DYING WITH CAROL

DYING WITH CAROL

BOB LILLIE

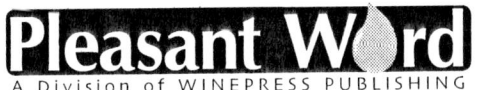
A Division of WINEPRESS PUBLISHING

© 2004 by Bob Lillie. All rights reserved.

Printed in the United States of America

Packaged by Pleasant Word, a division of WinePress Publishing, PO Box 428, Enumclaw, WA 98022. The views expressed or implied in this work do not necessarily reflect those of Pleasant Word, a division of WinePress Publishing. Ultimate design, content, and editorial accuracy of this work are the responsibilities of the author.

No part of this publication may be reproduced, stored in a retrieval system, or transmitted in any way by any means—electronic, mechanical, photocopy, recording, or otherwise—without the prior permission of the copyright holder, except as provided by USA copyright law.

Unless otherwise noted, all Scriptures are taken from the Holy Bible, New International Version, Copyright © 1973, 1978, 1984 by the International Bible Society. Used by permission of Zondervan Publishing House. The "NIV" and "New International Version" trademarks are registered in the United States Patent and Trademark Office by International Bible Society.

Scripture references marked KJV are taken from the King James Version of the Bible.

Scripture references marked NASB are taken from the New American Standard Bible, © 1960, 1963, 1968, 1971, 1972, 1973, 1975, 1977 by The Lockman Foundation. Used by permission.

ISBN 1-4141-0059-0
Library of Congress Catalog Card Number: 2003113577

TABLE OF CONTENTS

Chapter 1: The Early Experiences of This Couple through Cursillo and the Walk to Emmaus 7
Chapter 2: Discovering the Disease 11
Chapter 3: Early Surgery 23
Chapter 4: Chemo and Christmas 31
Chapter 5: Back to the Hospital 37
Chapter 6: The Second Surgery and Complications 41
Chapter 7: A Month in the Hospital 51
Chapter 8: Going Home with Hospice 71
Chapter 9: 49 Days with Hospice 79
Chapter 10: Carol's Funeral 191
Chapter 11: Bob's Thank You Sermon 207

Note from the Author 215

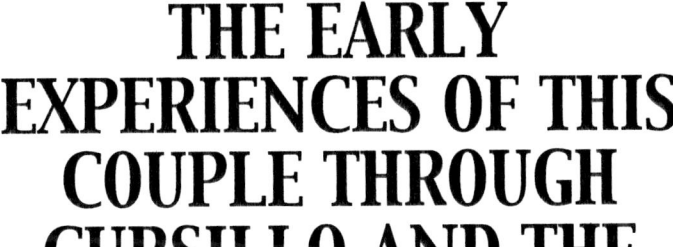

Chapter 1

THE EARLY EXPERIENCES OF THIS COUPLE THROUGH CURSILLO AND THE WALK TO EMMAUS

Even though we were married in 1955 and went to church every Sunday, we know now that we were not really Christians. We even took our children to Sunday school to try to raise them as Christians, but in many ways we didn't really understand the meaning of God's grace. I guess you could sum up my religious beliefs in the statement "do good things and you'll go to heaven, do bad things and you'll go to hell."

It wasn't until 1977, when one of my teachers, Marj Crowe, wanted to sponsor us to a Roman Catholic program called "Cursillo."

The Peoria Cursillo Community was one of the few Cursillo communities in the United States that allowed non-Catholics to attend. In August and September of 1977, I and then Carol attended Cursillo 117 and 119. In this movement husbands and wives go on different weekends. The husband always goes first. There was a cursillo in another city between our two walks.

The Cursillo movement started in Spain in the late 1940's to get men back into the life of the church. It came to the United States in 1957 when some Spanish air cadets, training in Texas, held a Cursillo weekend for a group of Spanish speaking men.

The first English language Cursillo was held in 1961 in San Angelo, Texas; that year, the movement spread to a dozen other states including Illinois.

The movement was introduced into the Peoria diocese in 1964, where it was ecumenical, open to all faiths.

In the early 80's the United Methodist Church out of Nashville, Tennessee wanted to start a version that they could use across the country, because few Roman Catholic Cursillo communities were ecumenical.

Because of a copyright of the Cursillo name and the fact that the national Roman Catholic Cursillo movement did not want it to be ecumenical, a new name was given to the United Methodist program: "Walk To Emmaus"

There were some changes to the program, but the general format of Cursillo was still followed.

The weekends consists of fifteen talks given by clergy and lay people and also some demonstrations by the Cursillo or Emmaus communities as to the real nature of God's undeserved love. In the Emmaus, it is called agape; in Cursillo it is called palanca.

Carol and I served on Cursillo teams and then eventually were asked to serve on the newly formed "Walk to Emmaus" teams. Because of the limited numbers in the beginning Walk to Emmaus community, we were generally asked to serve on a team once a year and sometimes twice.

The Early Experiences of This Couple through Cursillo and the Walk to Emmaus

We also became the registrars for the Central Illinois Walk to Emmaus community for five years.

What Cursillo and Walk to Emmaus did for us was to explain the real meaning of God's grace, that it was the undeserved, unearned love of God.

Finally, we knew that just doing "good works" did not buy you a ticket to heaven. What Jesus did on the cross, by dying for our sins was the thing that justified us and allowed us to face our God in a sinless state.

During our years of service in the Central Illinois Emmaus community, we were able to move up in leadership. Eventually, I was the lay director of Central Illinois Walk number 71 and Carol was the lay director of Central Illinois women's Walk number 99.

We also, during these years, served on Cursillo teams when we were called, and in September of 1999 I was asked to be a rector (lay leader) of men's Cursillo 606 in Peoria, Illinois. I consider this a great honor for a non-catholic to be invited to serve in this capacity.

After having served as lay directors in the Central Illinois Emmaus community, we no longer could serve on teams. They later changed that rule, but for a while we were not invited to serve. Because of this, and the fact that we had never served together, we decided to embark on a new ministry taking a similar type of program into the correctional facilities in Illinois. I was elected to the prison advisory board of "Faith, Hope, and Love" a prison ministry located in Peoria, Illinois.

We were able to serve together for the first time and had served on eleven prison teams and were scheduled to serve on our twelfth team, October 5, 2000.

Chapter 2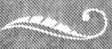

DISCOVERING THE DISEASE

August 14, 2000, Carol had a physical–heart, lungs, pelvic exam and a pap test. On Thursday, August 17 the pap test results came back all right. On September 13, she had a mammogram in a mobile unit and then on September 13 another mammogram at Methodist Hospital, along with a sonogram which found a small tumor. A needle biopsy determined it was a small grade 1 cancerous tumor in the very early stage. Wednesday September 20, we met with a breast cancer doctor where we were shown the x-ray and the tumor. Surgery was scheduled for October 5.

Carol started having some discomfort in the groin and stomach area and did not have any appetite. She complained to our family doctor who tested her for a urinary infection and took her off the lipitor she was taking.

On Monday September 25 she went to Methodist Hospital in Peoria for pre-testing for the surgery. We also met with the doctor who was going to oversee the radiation treatment. All of the doctors to this point thought Carol's protruding stomach was just gas.

On Wednesday, September 27, Carol had a very bad night. Her stomach was so bloated she could hardly turn over in bed.

I called our family doctor the next morning and was told to take Carol to the emergency room at Methodist Hospital.

We spent a total of seven hours in the E.R.

They put in an IV and took many x-rays. Finally, our family doctor ordered a CT scan. After they were finished they brought Carol back to the E.R.

Our doctor called and wanted to talk to me. I was told that Carol's ovary was enlarged and there were spots on her liver.

Carol was admitted to the hospital that night on the oncology floor. The nurse had a very difficult time putting in an IV and that caused a great deal of pain.

The next day they removed four and a half liters of fluid from her stomach cavity.

Carol's good friends, Jane Griffith and Ilona Mc Donough, both nurses, were waiting along with our pastor, Scott Carlson, when Carol came back to her room. She was now ten pounds lighter.

About 9:00 the next morning Dr. Brewers, an ovarian cancer doctor, came in and told us that she would do a hysterectomy. She was certain that the tumor in her left ovary was malignant and also the fatty sac near the ovary called momentum. She would also check the bowels, liver etc.

On Friday September 29, we took Carol home to wait for the October 5 surgery date. They would do both the breast surgery and the ovarian cancer surgery at the same time.

Discovering the Disease

During the ensuing weeks, Carol again filled up with cancerous fluid and was becoming very uncomfortable again.

Many of Carol's friends, her Walk to Emmaus reunion group and others came to pray with us and offer support during the week.

Our daughter-in law, Jennifer, sent our daughter, Robin, one of her frequent flyer tickets so that she could fly in from Phoenix, AZ to be there for her mother's surgery.

On October 5, we left for the hospital at 5:45 A.M. With me during the surgery would be our son Bob and his wife Jennifer, from southern Indiana, and our daughter Robin. Also present would be our good friends, Mary Jane and Roger Griffith, Ilona Mc Donough, our pastor, Scott Carlson, and our niece Tammy Graber. Also there were Robin's close friends Starr Shalk and Sherl Haag, Robin's in laws, Kay and Ralph Crow, who live in Illinois; Millard Day, a friend from the Walk to Emmaus, who is an employee of Methodist Hospital, and Joyce and Elton Lanier, a brother and sister-in law.

The breast lump was removed by one doctor, and then the ovarian cancer doctor took over for the next seven and a half hours. She was given a hysterectomy and also had a gallon of cancer fluid vacuumed out of her stomach cavity again. One of her bowels was like an accordion, the doctor told us, which made it very difficult to remove all of the fluid. We were told that there were also some spots on her liver.

The doctor told us after the surgery that one third of ovarian cancer patients respond to chemotherapy and have

Dying with Carol

at least five years; one third respond partially and can make it a year, the last third make it only about six months. I'm giving you this information so that you will better understand the next part of this account.

When this started, we went to our friends in our church, the Peoria Cursillo, and the Central Illinois Walk to Emmaus for prayer support.

I found that the easiest way to do this was to send almost daily e-mails to "Carol's Friends," the name of the file in my mailing list. This list grew as some of our friends started forwarding these daily messages to their Christian friends around the country.

I started sending these out on September 27. What follows is an almost daily log and many of the responses we received.

E-mail sent Wednesday, September 27, 2000 8:13 P.M.:

> Subject: Prayers needed for Carol
>
> I just got back from the emergency room at Methodist Hospital in Peoria. We were there since 10:00 A.M. Wednesday. They finally determined that Carol has a mass on her ovaries. We don't know if it is cancer yet, but the doctor suspects it is. There are also some spots on her liver. It doesn't sound good. We'll know more Thursday. She was to have her breast lump removed October 5.
>
> We need your prayers badly right now. She's in the Hamilton wing, Room 708

Discovering the Disease

Sent: Thursday, September 28, 2000, 10:18 P.M.:

Subject: Carol update

Carol has cancer of the ovaries and will have surgery, (we think) next Thursday October 5th. They will do both her breast surgery and her hysterectomy at the same time. She will have chemo after the surgery along with radiation. I will bring her home for a few days on Friday. She has been strong in her faith, relying on your prayers and God's mercy.

We love you all. Keep up the prayers.

Bob Lillie

The following e-mails were received September 29, 2000:

Bob & Carol,

We are Praying for you & Carol that God's healing touch will be felt by you both. Know that you are not alone– Thanks for the talk & as I give the talk on the weekend– you will be lifted up to the Lord– The team and pilgrims will be praying for you.

If there is anything more we can do, please do not hesitate to call us.

Love
Dick & Chris

Dying with Carol

Another e-mail from a friend Judi who is becoming a nun:

> Bob, I have requested all the sisters at the mother house to pray for Carol and you. We trust God for all things. You are in my heart and prayer.
>
> Love,
Judi

Dear Bob and Carol

Dick and I are in prayer for a marvelous healing for Carol. We are cursing that cancer at the root and commanding it to dry up just like the fig tree did when Jesus cursed it.

Be strong and of a good courage just like Joshua and you will enter your promised land.

Love to you both,
Dick and Beth Yost

Carol and Bob,

Our prayers are with you both. God is good, God is powerful, God is the only thing we need.

In His Service,
Terri Benz

Bob

Sorry to hear about Carol's diagnosis. We will continue to keep both of you in our prayers. If there is anything

Discovering the Disease

we can do for you let us know. Let us know what you find out. May god's blessings be with both of you.

Linnie

E-mails received September 30:

Hi Bob,

Received the prayer request for Carol. Please know that we are in prayer for both of you. You both hold a very special place in our hearts. Give Carol a hug for us and know that Our Creator is holding both of you in the palm of His hand.

Love,
Chuck & Dotty Fouse

Linda and I are praying for you and Carol and your family. If I can do anything to help, even if just to listen, please let me know.

Know you are loved,
Bruce

E-mail sent September 30 and the response:

Dr. Lynn Jalavec will remove a small tumor in Carol's breast. They will not take out the lymph nodes as is the usual procedure. When she is completed Dr. Cheryl Brewers will remove Carol's ovaries and give her a complete hysterectomy.

(I gave the doctor's names because I wanted our friends to pray for them also.)

Dying with Carol

E-mails received the next day, September 30:

Greetings Bob,

Continue to keep you and Carol in my prayers. I will add the Drs. to my list.

May you all experience God's peace thru all of this.

John

Bob

You know the old sports saying, "It is not over till the Fat Lady Sings."

Roger clued us in at the Walk meeting this morning and you were given to the prayer team. There will be a lot of us praying for you and Carol.

Hang in there man and if there is any way I can be of help, (I am already praying for you), let me know.

DeColores (a Cursillo and Emmaus greeting)

Roger

Dear Bob,

We are keeping you in prayer, that you would know the Lord's Strength in this difficult time. May God's presence be very evident in all of the friends and family that surround you. We love you.

Sue & John

Discovering the Disease

E-mail received October 1, 2000:

> Am continuing to pray for Carol as she faces these surgeries and results that the doctors will be guided by the hand of God and that nothing that is not of Him will be able to touch her. I also want to thank Carol for the encouraging hands that she sent to me as I was giving my 4th day talk today.
>
> I was overwhelmed when I read the things she wrote, knowing what she is going through and wanted to let her know what an inspiration and witness she was to me. I wasn't at the team meeting last week and as it turned out, they had just enough time for me to give my talk today. Know that you and your family are in my prayers although I'm not sure we've ever met, we have the strongest of bonds–Jesus Christ in whose name I pray for you, Carol, for healing and strength for you and your family.
>
> In His name,
Nancy Graf

Dear Bob and Carol,

Just wanted to let you know that Iris forwarded your info on Carol's surgery and treatment. You are both in my thoughts and prayers.

Love,
Dalene

Dying with Carol

Received e-mail October 2:

> Bob and Carol,
>
> We are lifting prayers of healing and restoration for you during this time in Carol's life. Praise God
> DeColores
>
> Lee and Linda Reffett

> Bob,
>
> You are both in our prayers, along with the doctors and your family.
>
> Sometimes trusting God is hard and yet it is during those times we must trust Him the most.
>
> God Bless,
Jeff & Kathern

E-mail received October 4:

> Bob & Carol
>
> May the Love of God that we all felt with you Bob, almost a year ago, and the Power God shared with all of us, in that Divine weekend spent with Cursillo #606 be some consolation to you and Carol in this time of God's Own Divine Plan!
>
> In our prayers,
Mark, Beth, Stephen, & David Seipel

Discovering the Disease

The following e-mails were received from someone we didn't know from the Walk to Emmaus chat room:

Robert and Carol

May you truly feel the presence of God as you walk through this valley of unknown. Our God is most merciful and gracious. May He guide you through these trials, and give you peace. Trust in Him with all your heart and soul and He will do the rest. May His Grace and Love sustain and keep you.

A sister and servant of Christ
Mary
Central Arizona

I will keep your wife in my prayers. My grandmother (God Bless Her) had breast cancer and ovarian cancer. May God surround the doctors, nurses, orderlies, and techs who will be with your wife with strength, courage, and healing hands. May God surround you and your wife with His peace, love, and strength. I will mention her at my Emmaus Reunion Group tonight. Take care. Let us know how she is doing.

Your newest sister in Him,
Nova Johnson

WTE
#61 Fort Worth Area Emmaus Lay Director

Dying with Carol

Here's another e-mail from someone we didn't know:

This is my prayer:

Heavenly Father: We praise you for you are the only and Almighty God and we are humbled by the knowledge that you love and care for each one of us.

At this time, I lift Carol to you. I boldly come before you as You have said that "if we ask, we shall receive." And so, I humbly ask that Dr. Brewers and Dr. Jalovec will be given wisdom, skill and direction in both of these surgeries that will be performed tomorrow. I pray that all of the cancer will be successfully removed and your grace and strength be given to Carol. Be with her husband at this time, giving him peace and grace during this difficult time. These are Your children and we know that you want the best for them. Thank you, Father, that we can come to you and lay our burdens and cares at your feet, that you hear and answer. In the precious name of Jesus, Amen.

God be with both of you.

In His love,
Lou Rogers

Bob,

I will be praying for your wife and the two surgeons. I had breast cancer surgery in August and am now having chemo. I know how important the prayers are.

Terry FL Crown Walk to Emmaus #29
Table of Esther

Chapter 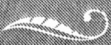 3

EARLY SURGERY

I sent out another general request for prayers October 4:

> On October 5 my wife, Carol Lillie, who was lay director of Central Illinois Walk #99 is going to have cancer surgery tomorrow, Thursday, October 5 at the Methodist Hospital in Peoria, Illinois. She has both breast cancer and ovarian cancer. She will have both surgeries tomorrow. She started in the movement with Cursillo in 1977 and has been involved in the Walk to Emmaus since 1985.
>
> I'm asking for prayers from all Emmaus pilgrims who receive this e-mail.
>
> Pray also for the two doctors Dr. Lynn Jalavec, who will do the breast surgery and Dr. Sheryl Brewers, who is doing the ovarian cancer surgery.
>
> In Jesus name,
> Bob Lillie

Dying with Carol

E-mail received October 5:

> Dear Mr. Lillie:
>
> I just wanted to assure you and your wife of my prayers as she undergoes surgery tomorrow. May the God of grace, the colors of which have shown so brightly through her involvement in Cursillo and Emmaus, shine even brighter in the recovery and healing God brings.
>
> Please know of my concern and desire for an update as you have opportunity.
>
> In Christ,
Ron Colwell, Director
The Upper Room Walk to Emmaus
>
> My prayers are with your wife and with you. Please keep me posted.
>
> May God keep you both.
>
> Vickie Caruthers
Charleston WV community

E-mail received October 6:

> Dear Robert,
>
> Know that members of the Keystone Emmaus Community are praying for you and your wife. May you feel God's healing presence as the days go by.
>
> Grace & Peace,
Brenda Eckert

Early Surgery

Dear Bob,

We have been praying for you and Carol daily. Even through the ordeal that I have been through in the past 2 weeks, we have asked God to not to let us forget others who are in need of prayer.

Prayer power is awesome.

I felt the power of all who prayed as they pushed me into the operating room. I told God I was ready if he wanted to take me now. I don't think I would be here right now if it weren't for all the prayers. He sent me back.

There are still things He wants me to do. I'm sure one of them is to pray for you and Carol. I will pray that she receives the same blessing that I received.

Our God is an awesome God.

Peace and love to you both
Harold and Carolyn Turner

Received October 10:

Please let Carol know that I am praying for both of you. I will never forget being on a team with her when she did the Study Talk, (I think that was the one) and talked about Stick a Geranium in Your Hat and Be Happy. I have shared that book with so many people since then and I have always been grateful to Carol for introducing me to it. I continue to pray that both of you find that pain is inevitable but misery is optional and for the

Dying with Carol

chemo to work and for Carol to be able to continue her strong Christian witness.

DeColores
Ann Russell
CIE Walk #37

Sent: Wednesday, October 11, 2000 5:24 P.M.:

Subject: Carol Lillie up-date after surgery
Carol Lillie, Peoria Cursillo 118 in 1977
Lay Leader Central Illinois Emmaus Walk #99
To all of our Cursillo and Walk to Emmaus friends:

Two days ago I asked for prayers for my wife who was to undergo surgery for both breast and ovarian cancer at the Methodist Hospital in Peoria, Illinois.

The response from our friends (known and unknown) has been overwhelming.

It has been almost like the Palanca or agape letters we get when we are on a Cursillo or Walk to Emmaus.

I would like to up-date what has happened in the last twenty-four hours and ask for your continued prayers.

Carol spent seven and a half hours in surgery on Thursday. The first hour the breast lump was removed and then the second surgeon took over and started on the ovarian cancer. They did a hysterectomy and removed a large tumor from one of her ovaries. The other one was also infected. There was cancer attached to part of her

Early Surgery

intestine and her bladder that they tried to vacuum out. They believe they got most of it.

I spent the night with her and with medication she has now, she does not have a lot of pain. Her mouth is very dry and she is living on ice chips and IV's.

What I want you to pray about now is that the chemotherapy that they will start in 8 to 10 days will be effective in reducing a blood C.A. 125 count down to a acceptable number.

God has brought us through the surgery and now with God's help, medical science will grant my wife of 45 years a longer productive life.

I also ask for your prayers for a group of Christians who are taking a similar program into the Dwight Correctional Center in Dwight, Illinois this weekend.

Carol was going to be a table leader, and I was going to be in the Agape (Palanca) chapel and give the Talk, "God Is Love."

Thanks again for your support.

Bob Lillie
Eureka, Illinois

Received October 16:

    Bob and Carol

    Thanks for keeping us informed of Carol's prayer needs. Know she is held up to the throne from where all grace and mercy and healing comes. I just sent a card off this morning, and Bob, thank you for the posters. I shared with the team how you so graciously offered them to me when I was hoping I didn't need to use them, and you didn't know you wouldn't be back. I did need them and they worked great . . . . And if God cares about posters . . . believe me He cares about the hurts his children face and will see things are taken care of.

Love and Prayers,
Violet

Dear Bob and Carol,

As you enter the time of uncertainty with Chemo, know that we are praying for the medicine that only our Maker could allow us to create would do its work and kill any remaining cancer cells. We pray for strength and courage for both of you that you may be a comfort to each other and that you can also draw on each other's strength that only the Holy Spirit can supply us with.

We ask that Carol will have the strength to be a witness to others with whom she comes in contact and that the Lord might be glorified through that and that He pour out His mercy and grace upon both of you.

Nancy and Karl Graf

Dear Robert and Carol,

A little over four years ago my wife and I also experienced the testing of that time when you hear the words ovarian cancer. We were fortunate in that Pam's cancer

Early Surgery

was found in a relatively early stage during an operation to repair a problem with her colon. We're praying that the Lord will comfort and heal you during this time.

DeColores,
Tom and Pam

Chapter 4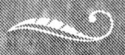

CHEMO AND CHRISTMAS

Bob wrote on Tuesday October 17:

> We just got back from Carol's first chemo treatment. It took 6 hours of IV's, but she hasn't (so far) experienced any adverse reactions. They give a lot of anti-nausea medicine and they also sent home two prescriptions, one for nausea and one a sedative to be taken before she goes to bed.
>
> The last two nights, she has been coming upstairs to sleep in her own bed; she still uses the hospital bed we have in the living room during the day, but she sleeps better in her own bed.
>
> Dr. Brewers told her that her CA125 count was 415 before the surgery. It has dropped to 146 now because of the removing the cancer cells during the surgery. Dr.

Dying with Carol

Brewers said our goal was to get it down to under 35 after the chemo.

They will be testing for it to see how much good the chemo is doing. The doctor did come in and check her heart and lungs to make sure the chemo wasn't having any adverse reactions. All was good. Pray that she doesn't get sick in the next 48 hours. Thanks again for your prayers. We have received 106 e-mails from around the country from our Emmaus and Cursillo family.

Love,
Bob

E-mail received October 18:

Praise the Lord!

God is good! Have been thinking of the two of you much lately. I will share this praise with the two prayer chains I sent the original prayer request to.

We will continue with prayers,

In His name,
Eva Marie
Walk #76 (Apostolic Center)

Dear Bob and Carol,

Just a quick note to tell you that you are ever in our prayers. Persevere, dear friends.

Chemo and Christmas

Our friend Carol Broyles is undergoing aggressive chemo for breast cancer, just started Tuesday. I gave her your name Carol and she prays for you. She is a Cursillo friend from Tryo Mo.

Love,
Jon and Mary Jane Davis

October 23, sent this e-mail:

Thank you for your prayers.

We want to thank all of our friends from the Eureka United Methodist Church and the Eureka and Woodford County community for all of their prayers for Carol. During her surgery and recuperation from breast and ovarian cancer, the response has been overwhelming. Carol has received over 135 get-well cards and over 140 e-mails from our Walk to Emmaus and Cursillo communities across the country, as well as friends and relatives.

We feel that your prayers have already been answered because although Carol had to go through seven and a half hours of major surgery and six hours of chemotherapy, she has not had a great deal of pain and very little sickness from the chemotherapy.

We are asking that you keep her in your prayers during the following six months of chemotherapy and that the treatment will be successful in freeing her from cancer.

We will pray for you all and we know with God's help, His will, will be done.

Dying with Carol

God has blessed us through you.

> Carol and Bob Lillie
> Eureka, Illinois

During the time between Carol's October chemotherapy and the next e-mail in January, Carol was somewhat tired, but we had some good time at home. At Christmas, we had our daughter, Robin, and our grandchildren, Aaron and Acacia, at home and also our son, Bob and his wife Jennifer.

Our grandchildren, from Arizona, had a ball with all of the snow we had on the ground. Even though it was quite cold, they went sledding several times. This was a new experience for kids who were born and raised in Phoenix, Arizona.

Carol did take a nap each afternoon, but for the most part it was one of the best family Christmas's we have had.

God did provide both a reprieve in Carol's illness and the opportunity for the family to all to be here. We know, of course, that Carol's cancer was the reason the family made the financial sacrifice to be here this year.

We continued on with chemotherapy at three-week intervals until the end of January when the next e-mail was sent.

January 22, 2001

We got home about 1:00 P.M. from Carol's chemo and she went straight to bed. She did get sick some, but not as much as she did last week. I've got to give her a shot

Chemo and Christmas

each night for five nights to build up her blood count to protect her from infections. Last time it took 3 days before she felt better. At least she doesn't have another chemo treatment for 3 weeks. She does have to get a blood test in ten days. Pray that this treatment lowers her CA125 count.

>Love to all,
>Bob Lillie

Her CA125 count is a cancer marker that can tell whether or not the chemotherapy is working. Unfortunately, it can't be used to detect ovarian cancer. As of now there is no test that can look for early signs of this cancer.

January 24 2001, e-mail just to our children:

> Your mother has spent the last two days in bed and hasn't eaten hardly anything. I went to the doctor's in Peoria and got another anti-nausea pill for her to take. I've been giving her a shot each day for her blood count; I hope she feels better tomorrow.
>
>>Dad

Received January 25 from Robin, our daughter, and a note returned:

> Tell her we love her and we're praying for her. Keep me posted. I love you.
>
>>Robin

She's a little better this morning. She ate some cream of wheat and got some of her new anti-nausea pills down. Just pray that this will reduce her CA125 count.

Love,
Dad

January 27, e-mail sent to our son and his wife Jennifer:

We got the flowers this morning and they are beautiful. Mom was stronger yesterday, but still not up to her regular self. We finished the last shot injection this morning to raise her blood count. She goes for a blood test Wednesday and a CA125 February 7th. The next chemo is February 15th.

Thanks again,
Dad

As you will see from the next e-mails, this schedule did not materialize.

Chapter 5
BACK TO THE HOSPITAL

Sunday January 28, 12:45 our time:

Mom's still not eating much and in bed. The doctor said to call and get an appointment for Monday if she isn't better by then. I'll keep you posted.

Dad

Monday January 29

I'm taking Mom to see Dr. Brewers at 2:30 P.M. today. I'll let you know how things turn out. I almost hope she'll put her in the hospital for tests.

Dad

Tuesday January 30 sent out to all of "Carol's Friends":

Ever since her last chemo on Monday the 22nd, Carol hasn't eaten hardly anything and her blood count is way down. Yesterday, I took her to Dr. Brewers and she immediately put her in Methodist Hospital. She's on IV's and antibiotics to fight off an infection. She has a bowel blockage that is a result of the original tumor or severe constipation. We are hoping for the latter. The doctor says she will be in the hospital 5 to 7 days.

Her room number is Hamilton wing, room 721.

Bob

Subject: Wednesday Carol up-date
Date: Wed, Jan 31, 2001, 4:04 P.M.

Carol still hasn't eaten anything. She's on IV's, but they are cutting down on them to see if she will start eating. We are praying that her bowel blockage will open up. There were some encouraging signs yesterday. If they don't, she may have to have a colostomy. Her original ovarian cancer tumor was wrapped around a bowel.

The good news today is her white blood cell count came up to almost normal.

Her platelets are still very low. They may have to give her a transfusion. They want to get her blood count up high enough so they can put a medi-port under her skin so she can have chemo and draw blood without sticking her every time. It took six sticks and three blow-outs before they got her IV in on Monday.

We don't know how long she will be in Methodist Hospital in Peoria. I've been staying with her all night. She

Back to the Hospital

didn't sleep much Monday night or Tuesday. She was sleeping a lot today.

Keep praying for both of us.

Bob

(Note the Peoria hospital is 22 miles from Eureka, a 44-mile round trip)

Thursday February 1 at 3:45 P.M.

Just got back from the hospital to clean up. I'm going right back. With the help of a pain shot, Carol slept well Wednesday night. She still isn't eating anything to speak of. They were going to start giving her enemas today to clear out the blockage. Her blood count has improved so they may do the shunt things before she leaves. The doctor is still talking about a permanent colostomy if the bowel stays restricted.

Another friend from church came in this afternoon so I could come home and clean up. I don't know when she'll get to come home.

Hanging in there,
Bob

Friday February 2, 2001

They put a shunt into Carol today so that they don't have to stick her any more for IV's, chemo, or to draw blood. It took two tries this morning at 5:30 A.M. to get blood for a blood test. She still is not eating very much.

Dying with Carol

I'm afraid they may have to do the colostomy, if she doesn't pass food through pretty soon. She'll be in the hospital at least to the beginning of next week.

She is in no pain, but her stomach is constantly upset. She is sleeping well now with the help of medication.

Love to all.
Bob

Sat., February 3, 2001, 1:17 P.M.

Carol will have surgery for a bowel blockage Sunday morning at about 10:00 A.M. They're going to tap her lung this afternoon. Pray for Dr. Brewers and us.

The outlook for the future is in God's hands.

Bob

Chapter 6

THE SECOND SURGERY AND COMPLICATIONS

Sunday February 4

Carol had surgery Sunday to repair both small and large intestines that were blocked by her ovarian cancer. They also did a colostomy so that she would not have this problem again. Tonight (Sunday 8:00 P.M.) she is resting without pain in the intensive care ward of Methodist Hospital. She will probably stay in the cancer ward (Hamilton) for approximately a week.

We did get some better news because her CA125 (cancer count) numbers did go down this week to 150. That means the chemo is doing some good. The doctor is planning to give her another chemo treatment before she leaves the hospital.

Please keep us and the doctors in your prayers.

Bob

Dying with Carol

Tuesday February 6

As I said yesterday, Carol came through the bowel blockage surgery all right, but there is also fluid around her right lung. This morning the doctor said it was partially collapsed and the good lung has a small amount of fluid in it (pneumonia). The doctor thinks the antibiotics will take care of that, but this morning at 5:00 A.M. and x-ray crew accidentally pulled out the tube from her nose and after 6 failed attempts by nurses, Dr. Brewers finally got it restored. It drains fluid from her stomach. This poor girl has been through so much, but her faith is strong and she knows how to smile.

I thank God for her trust.

Bob

E-mail received February 6:

Bob:

I love you guys. I hope you both know that. As best you can, give Carol a hug from me and tell her that I love her and am praying for her. Then have Roger or someone close at hand give you a hug for me.

Shalom
Bruce

Wednesday February 7, 2001, from Bob:

The Second Surgery and Complications

The good news is that the doctor said that Carol is healing well from her surgery and her partially deflated lung is working better and filling up with air.

Carol, however, has gone through so much these last few weeks that she is in almost a psychotic state. The doctor assures me this is just temporary because of a chemical imbalance in her body, but it is very frightening to us when she doesn't recognize us or her friends. Last night she was repeating the same phrases over and over again. I could get her to say the Lord's Prayer and the twenty-third psalm with me and sing "Jesus Loves Me." Today she isn't saying anything at all. Pray that her chemistry gets straightened out and she gets back to her own loving self.

Bob

E-mail received February 8:

Carol has really been thru it all this past year and still. I will be praying for her Bob, we all know God does answer prayer. And how are you holding up thru all of this? You too, are in my prayers, so that the love of God will touch the both of you, comfort you and give you peace.

Love,
Kathern

E-mail received February 9:

Dying with Carol

Dear Bob,

Just wanted you to know that you and Carol were lifted up in prayers at 1st United Methodist Church choir tonight (in Peoria). You must be exhausted beyond belief.

With love,
Kassin

Another e-mail received February 8:

Somehow or another I just erased all that I had written, so will start over. You don't know me personally, I'm not sure we've ever met, but I wanted to tell you and Carol how much you mean to me and how you've touched my life. I was the first team member on the team that Carol was supposed to be on last fall. I still have the hands that she cut out and were laying at my place, encouraging me in giving my first "4th day" talk. When I heard that she was sick and my friend Marilyn Goddard was taking her place, I couldn't believe that she had taken the time, with all of her personal concerns, to write those notes. After all this time, I now understand. Just from the updates that you send and from the things that Mary Jane (Griffith) and that Marilyn says, I know that both of you are very special people whom God is using in a special way.

I continue to pray for you both that he will continue to use you and to give you the strength, courage, and comfort that you need when you need it.

I also continue to pray for healing for her and will until God tells me only to pray for peace.

The Second Surgery and Complications

I wanted you both to know how you have touched my life and I'm sure the lives of many others.

My prayers for both of you continue. May Jesus wrap his loving arms around you and let you feel the reality of His touch.

I thank God that both of you are in my life.

Nancy Graf

I sent this e-mail February 8:

Subject: Keep prayers coming

This morning (Thursday) they did an EEG (brain wave) and determined Carol had not had a seizure. They have given her something so that after three days, she is finally closing her eyes and sleeping for a short period of time, but then her arm and leg twitching begins all over. She does keep her eyes closed. The doctor still thinks she had a rare reaction to one of her drugs. They were considering a brain scan, but as of now, she isn't still enough to do a cat scan. The doctor sent me home for a day to rest and Jane Griffith and Audrey Lasswell are staying with her. I'll go back around five P.M.

She hasn't recognized me for two days now. I pray that after she gets some sleep she will. The one thing that keeps me going is your prayers. I can really feel them.

Bob

Dying with Carol

E-mail received February 9:

> Almighty and Holy God,
>
> I pray that you will bless Carol with healing and peace of mind. I also ask that you comfort Robert and the rest of the family. You, O Lord, are the maker of miracles and I believe you will work a miracle in Carol and her family. I believe that you will reveal to them your wonderful love, grace, and majesty. To you I give honor, praise, and glory in the powerful name of Jesus. AMEN.

Sent: Saturday, February 10, 2001 8:35 P.M.:

> Subject: Saturday Carol prayer report
>
> I didn't make it home yesterday because the weather report scared me to think I might not make it back to the hospital. Our son, Bob, and his wife, Jennifer drove in from Louisville, KY and are spending the night with Carol so that I can sleep in my bed for the first time this week. My prayers were answered when Carol recognized Bob at once when he spoke to her. She keeps her eyes closed most of the time, but she is getting better at times in responding to us. We got some good news yesterday that her MRI of the brain did not show any cancer, so we are working on an unusual medication reaction as the cause of her problem. Her white blood cell count is going down so she is fighting any infection she might have.
>
> The doctor said today we would be at Methodist Hospital for a week or 10 days if all goes well.

The Second Surgery and Complications

Thank you for your many prayers.

Bob

(I ran into Rev. Tom Eckhart in the hall last night on the cancer floor. His mother-in law had just died.)

Received Sunday February 10:

Dear Bob,

So glad to hear your son could come and relieve you for one night. Dear heart, you must be exhausted. I know how it is to see a loved one under so much medication that they cannot think straight. My dad was like that for awhile. He thought he was fishing in Minnesota, while in a bed at St. Mary's. It does pass as the medication is relaxed. Glad to hear some good news of Carol's MRI and white count. You both are in my prayers, daily. I even have the teachers at school praying each Tues. morning.

Bob, please pray that I can do God's work as Lay Director on the women's walk in May. I finally said yes . . and am scared that I won't hear who He is calling.

God's Peace to you both,

Love,
Judy McKinney

Dying with Carol

Also received February 11:

Bob

I am so glad that Carol recognized you. I know that made you feel so much better. I am glad that Bob and Jennifer are here to help. I hope you slept well. You are in my prayers throughout the day.

Love Ya!
Marj

Subject: Two weeks in the hospital and still counting
Date: Monday, Feb 12, 2001, 2:03 P.M.

I don't know how many of our friends, who have been receiving my e-mails about Carol's battle with ovarian cancer, watched "Touched By An Angel" Sunday night. (Carol was not aware of the show.)

The mother in the story was facing a very uncertain future with the reoccurrence of ovarian cancer. The husband, a science teacher, did not believe in God and didn't want his daughter to believe in God.

For the first time since Carol's ordeal started I found myself in tears. (Men don't cry; their eyes sweat.) I was crying because of something Carol had said when we first found out she had cancer. She wondered how anyone could possibly face this kind of problem without a belief in an all-powerful God, who loves us.

In last night's story the father with the help of angels discovered that God does exist. Both Carol and I believe

The Second Surgery and Complications

that He is watching over us, no matter what happens. We have been sustained by your prayers and we know that with them, the love of our friends, and the power of the Holy Spirit; God's will "will be done."

Thank you for your love and concern.

Bob

Chapter 7

A MONTH IN THE HOSPITAL

Sent: Tuesday, February 13, 2001 1:12 P.M.:

Subject: The doctors say things are improving

Two of Carol's doctors this morning said that Carol's awareness is improving. It may be hard for me to see because I am with her most of the time. She pulled the nose tube out that was draining her stomach last night before I could stop her. The doctor decided to let it out so that is a step in the right direction. Sandy and Paul Walles (our previous pastor and his wife) stopped in from Canton, Illinois and Carol seemed to recognize them. They are still working on the mystery that sent Carol into this psychosis after her surgery. Her mind is going continually, except when she is asleep, but she doesn't make much sense most of the time. She did repeat the Lord's Prayer with me today.

Dying with Carol

If it wasn't for this setback, we would probably be home by now from the surgery.

God bless you all for your prayers and concern for both of us.

Bob

Received February 13:

Bob,

I just wanted to send a note to tell you we are praying very hard for Carol and the family. Mom has been keeping me informed on a daily basis. Don't wear yourself out, I know it's hard not to, Carol will need you in good health when she comes home. Reading your letters and updates every day has been a real testament of faith to me. God bless you and Carol. We love you both!

Dave and Family
(Dave Blunier is our nephew)

Bob sent this February 14:

Last night Carol's nurse took it upon herself to cut Carol's night time medication in half. She only got one hour of sleep and I didn't get any. When I talked to the doctor this morning, he checked the charts and acknowledged that she did and said he would make the orders even clearer for her. I tried to tell the nurse at midnight, but I wasn't sure whether the doctor had changed the orders. This morning he assured me he did not.

A Month in the Hospital

I really feel we are under attack by evil powers. Carol's surgery is improving fine, but her mental state is frightening to me. I'm starting to better understand the demons they talked about in the Bible. When Carol was "with us" yesterday she asked for her Bible although, I know at present she can't read it.

Please pray, "In the name of Jesus" leave Carol and make her well.

Received February 15:

I pray in concert with you–you harassing spirits, you spirits that have moved in that room. I command you to leave in the name of Jesus. The room and the equipment and all that is in there I pray that the blood of Jesus cover. That it, cover Carol and Bob and anyone who enters that room. If anything is clinging to the Dr.'s or the nurses, I command that you remain outside that room as the doorway and any windows are covered by the blood.

I take authority over any spirits of anxiety, pain, harassment and anyones that are there that I can't name right now and in the name of Jesus and the power of His blood and the Victory on the Cross I take authority over you and I bind, fetter and gag you and send you to the place that Jesus has prepared for you, never to return.

Bob, you can copy this and take it to Carol's room and repeat these same things if you would like. We have the authority given by Jesus to do this. First, cover yourself with the armor.

Dying with Carol

I pray this prayer for both of you. Karl and I are attending a school on prayer for deliverance and healing and this is part of what we do. You, being in the room may discern some spirits that I don't from here–the spirit of fear, etc. might be one. Cover yourself and Carol with the glorious, victorious Blood. Satan thinks he's winning, well he isn't.

> Love of Christ to both of you,
> Nancy Graf

Also received from a past minister of our church:

Bob,

I know what you mean. This is spiritual warfare. We have been there. We're praying that Satan gets his hands off God's property.

> Danny

Bob wrote February 15:

Carol had a good night's sleep with the proper medication. It is so frustrating to see, although her body is recovering nicely from the surgery, her mind is in another world. She is really baffling the doctors. The geriatric psychiatrist is going to eliminate another one of her medications, but he admits he hasn't seen anything like this before.

I am so grateful for my church friends and my Emmaus who have been coming every afternoon to spell me for a few hours so I can get home, clean up, and write these e-mails, and get some rest.

A Month in the Hospital

Carol needs constant supervision. She would not be able to ring for a nurse if she knew what she needed. Her eye-hand coordination would not allow her to find the call button. She is very confused and we are not always sure if she recognizes us or not. She will repeat something like the "Lord's Prayer," if you say it with her. They're going to put another tube in her to feed her in the stomach rather than through her veins.

I was looking through her Bible this morning and I found a note on healing, about having the elders of the church anoint her with oil. I'll ask our pastor and some church elders to do that.

Thank you again for all
of your prayers,
Bob

Also received February 15:

Bob,

I was talking to Father Tim last night and found out he is unaware of Carol's illness. He is pastor at St. Joseph Church in Pekin. He has a new e-mail address since he is not with Cursillo any longer. I gave him a brief overview of Carol's situation but I'm sure he would like to hear from you directly.

We are continuing to pray for Carol and all your family. God Bless.

John & Darlene Wood

Dying with Carol

Friday February 16

My Dear Friends in Christ,

Carol has been in the hospital 19 days now and the end is not in sight. She had a good night last night and slept (with the aid of medication) most of the night. She still has the doctors baffled as to what is causing her psychotic condition.

They are now looking at some kind of an infection and are treating her again with antibiotics (different ones this time).

She does respond to us and knows us, but her speech is confused and many times unintelligible.

When I left to come home for a few hours today they had her sitting up in a chair. We did get some good news from the doctor that her CA125 (cancer) count has come down to 124 from 170. That means the chemo she had on January 22 is working to some degree.

It is really difficult to see someone you love in such a confused condition. If you have any family member who has had a stroke, you would understand what I mean; although the doctors still keep saying it is not a stroke.

I thank you for all your prayers for both of us.

Bob

A Month in the Hospital

Received February 17:

Bob,

Thanks for the updates on Carol. Just wanted you to know about ten years ago I had a serious liver problem which caused a chemical imbalance in my body. I was in the hospital for a little more than three weeks. Chuck can really identify with what you are going through as I was in a confused state as well.

Know that we are diligently praying for you and wisdom for the doctors to get to the bottom of Carol's confusion problem.

Love,
Dotty (& Chuck) Fouse

Bob wrote Saturday February 17:

Dear Friends of Prayer,

Carol slept the whole night through for the first time in weeks. I kept waiting for her to wake up so I could call the nurse for another shot, but she slept from 9:00 P.M. until 7:00 A.M. I really expected her to be improved mentally after that, but she is still in a state as if she had a mild stroke. The doctors are now thinking that may be a possibility even though the tests don't seem to indicate it.

Our pastor, Scott Carlson, did a healing anointing. He asked Carol if she wanted him to do it and she did answer with a very distinct, "Yes."

Dying with Carol

This morning, however, she still is constantly trembling in the arms and legs and speaks unintelligibly.

I'm usually in her room from 5:00 P.M. until about noon the next day, when someone spells me. We can't leave her alone because she wouldn't be able to ring for the nurse if she knew she needed one.

Tuesday night, Margo Tennis is going to spend the night so I can sleep in my own bed. I've been up there all but two nights. My son stayed a week ago today and on February 4th, she was in the ICU after her surgery.

I really want to thank everyone who takes the time to read these daily e-mails. I think it does me good just to sum up each 24 hours and share it with people I know who care.

Love to all,
Bob

Received Saturday February 17:

My dear brother in Christ

I appreciate very much that you keep me posted about Carol. In fact I open my e-mail to see if I have received a update. I shall continue to fast two more days. As I told you in a previous e-mail, I was going to for 4 days.

If we only knew God's plan in all of this.

I really believe that all things work for good to those who love God and are called to his purpose. I have kept

A Month in the Hospital

Florence Day posted also and she is our community prayer warrior, and she knows both you and Carol.

Know you are both thought of and prayed for by many people whom you do not even know. My roommate Judy for instance . . . I read your updates to her every day also.

Your Sister in Christ,
Julie Sechrest

Bob wrote Sunday February 18:

My Dear Friends of Prayer,

My thoughts turn this morning to the parable of the persistent widow in the 18th chapter of Luke. It is a story of persistence in prayer. For three weeks now Carol has been in Methodist Hospital and hundreds of you have been praying for her recovery. She has shown some improvement, but 21 days in a hospital with IV's and tubes running into her is a long time.

I hope none of you are getting discouraged in asking for Carol's healing. You may wonder how I can keep sending these e-mail messages almost each day, but sitting next to her bed each night, I feel so helpless and this is the one thing I can do for her, to ask all of our many Christian friends to be persistent in asking for God's healing.

Carol always told me of my impatience and now I have had to learn to wait on God's time.

Dying with Carol

Love to all,
Bob

Received Sunday February 18:

Dear Bob,

We do continue to pray for healing and will as long as God tells us to.

He says to ask, and one translation has in parentheses that it means to keep asking. We are to be persistent and will continue to be. Know that the prayers of the people of God are with you both. We pray that you may get adequate rest so that you can continue to be there for her as you have been.

And I thank God for Marilyn and Mary Jane and the rest of her friends and your family who have helped in that endeavor.

Love in Christ,
Nancy Graf

Bob wrote February 19:

My Dear Friends of Prayer,

When I left the hospital at noon, Sue Ewan as well as Audrey Lasswell were with Carol. Carol was especially glad to see Sue because she came all the way from Branson, Missouri to see her. Sue is now an associate United Methodist minister. Carol and I feel we had a little something to do with that because we sponsored Sue and John through the "Walk to Emmaus" several

A Month in the Hospital

years ago, which lead to Sue retiring from being a school teacher and into the full time ministry.

When I left, Sue was talking to Carol about heaven and bringing her a sense of peace that I could not do.

What we are hoping for now is that Carol will get strong enough to spend some time at home, but that's in God's hands.

Please keep up with your prayers. So far Carol has not experienced any pain, but her inability to speak clearly is very frustrating for her. They still can't tell if she has had a mild stroke or if something else is causing her confusion.

One thing she is not confused about is her love for Jesus and her family.

Love to all,
Bob

Bob wrote February 20:

Things are progressing with Carol slow, but sure. The highlight of my day was when she said, "Bob, water." That was the first time on her own she asked for something. She had a good night Monday night so we both got some sleep.

We had a rehabilitation doctor come in and check her today so hopefully in a few days she'll move to a rehabilitation room. We also had a speech therapist check to see if she could swallow properly, but I guess that is still a few days off.

Dying with Carol

It is still a mystery as to whether she had a stroke or something else is causing her psychosis. I thank the Lord for all of my Christian friends for their prayers and help.

One thing I have learned is that we, as Christians, must be good receivers of his love and grace. We want to do good for others and that is fine, but we also must put aside our pride (which is an obstacle to grace) and be able to accept the free undeserved gift from God and God's people. Over the last weeks, I have learned about how to be a receiver and not just a giver.

God bless you all,
Bob

Bob received February 20:

Bob,

I don't want to take much of your time . . . I know it's limited when you're home . . . but I wanted to let you know that Steve and I continue to keep Carol, you and your family in our prayers. I await your updates daily and pray for the needs that become apparent in every report you give.

God's time is hard to understand, I know, and it's even harder to wait upon. But He is good. You know that. Carol knows that.

Hang in there, Dear Brother. Your brothers and sisters in Christ are with you.

Trish Caldwell
CIE Walk #16

A Month in the Hospital

Received February 21:

Hi Bob,

I'm so sorry things don't seem to get better, but keep e-mailing. Sometimes just by sitting down and writing, it seems to ease some of the burden at least for me it does.

I'm still praying for Carol, we just have to believe that God will heal Carol and we have to stand on God's word and His promises that He has given us as his children.

He tells us that disease comes from Satan, so we have to bind Satan in prayer and ask that Carol be released from him, so that God can come in and heal. Yes, sometimes we just have to "Be Still and know that He is God." I'm not very good at agreeing with God's time table on things, but I guess I just have to trust Him.

Love,
Kathern

February 22 Bob wrote:

After 24 days, what do you pray for? My wife Carol is not getting better. First breast cancer, then ovarian cancer, then a bowel blockage, from the ovarian cancer, two surgeries, and now the doctors said she has probably had a slight stroke. Carol knows what is happening to her, but her speech is very limited and she doesn't seem to have much control of her muscles in her arms or legs.

What should we pray for? Perfect healing that will come from a new body with the Lord?

Dying with Carol

On Monday when Sue Ewan was here, Sue asked me if I had told Carol that she could go. I had not! On Tuesday night when Margo Tennis, a person who taught nursing at Illinois Weslyan University, was here, Carol's breathing became labored and, thank God, Margo knew what to tell the nurses what to do so that Carol survived. I know that was God's hand was protecting Carol. When things looked pretty grim that night Margo asked Carol if she should call me, but Carol said, "No, Bob needs to get some sleep." With all of her problems, she was thinking of me.

It is doubtful that Carol will get better. What then should we pray for? When you see her with tubes up her nose to feed her, another tube to help her breath, two devices to remove waste products from her, you can picture what her life is like now.

We know her life with Jesus will be so much better.

What should we pray for? My daughter told me the other day that she is praying that when I die, it will be swift, and I thanked her for that. That's real love!

I'm going to lie down now for a few hours before I go back to the hospital.

Pray that God's will, "will be done."

Love to all,
Bob

A Month in the Hospital

Received February 22:

My Dear Friend Bob,

I can't find words to really reply to your post. My heart breaks for all of you. I feel that I should share a part of my Catholic tradition with you. When I was a young girl, I was taught that St. Joseph was the Patron of a Happy Death. It was believed that to die surrounded by the love of your family and in the presence of Jesus was the perfect way to die. I did not really understand this until my adulthood. I have always been pretty direct–going straight to my Creator when I have a need. However, I do find comfort in asking St. Joseph to become part of the Prayer Chain praying for perfect healing for Carol.

May the Saints (those canonized and those known only in our hearts) join hands with all those who know and love Carol and Bob as we pray to know and accept God's will in all things.

Love Ya!
Marj

I answered Marj:

Thank you Marj, that really helped.

Bob sent this Friday February 23:

Carol's condition

We spent the night aspirating Carol every hour (or less) for fluids that are building up in her throat and lungs. I

Dying with Carol

sat down with the doctor this morning. On Monday, we will make a decision as to whether we should contact hospice and allow Carol to go home for her final days. (note: Carol and I were both Stephen's ministers in our church so we were both aware of what going home with hospice means.)

I thought a lot about it last night as I sat there in her darkened room and heard her labored breathing.

I'm still not giving up on a great miracle, but I'm thinking that Carol would be so much better off with our Heavenly Father than struggling for breath in a hospital room.

I'm not sure (as is no one) how long she will last at home, but I am sure she would be happiest in the house that she loved. Our friends from the church and Emmaus have been so faithful and comforting, I know I would not be able to get through this without their help.

God does provide angels in human form.

In His Love,
Bob

Received February 24:

Robert,

Without using names, I shared this e-mail with some minister friends of mine. Please allow me to share their thoughts.

A Month in the Hospital

You obviously already know that there are no easy answers in this case. It seems that when things are moving along fairly smoothly, life at large has a tendency to direct us over some bumpy paths without much warning. When we don't know what to pray, we should simply ask God to send the Holy Spirit so
that the groaning of our hearts can be interpreted as prayer, then pray the hardest prayer that will ever come out of our hearts and mouths.

Pray that God's will would be done. The first thing I would pray for is not a request, but a thanksgiving–for all the good things that come out of misery, for all the good things shared when the sun was shining and before the clouds came, for all the impact that the loved one has had on friends and family members, for the good memories of their life together. Then I would pray for peace and comfort for the sick and their loved ones, and finally, I would ask for understanding. I pray for these things for your friend, and I offer thanksgiving for your caring and support.

Robert, I know a tough decision is coming Monday. I pray that God will give you strength and comfort. Honestly, I don't know what else to ask for. A miracle would be great and marvelous. But through it all God is there; God is awesome; God is good–all the time.

Brother Clayton

Dying with Carol

Received Sunday February 25:

Bob,

I can't tell you how much it has meant to be kept informed with your daily letters. I would respond more often but I know that you don't have much time and I don't want you to feel obligated to read and or respond back when your time could be better spent resting. Please know that our thoughts and prayers are with you.

Love,
Patty

Bob sent Sunday February 25:

I'm home from the hospital to go to church. Our niece, Tammy Graber, is at the hospital with Carol, now so I can go to church and then get some rest.

Carol has a new problem. The stroke has made her so that she cannot swallow at all. If we try to feed her through her mouth the food might choke her, or go into her lungs. They are now feeding her through a tube in her nose directly into her stomach. I don't know how we will feed her if we get her home. I hope hospice has some ideas. She is still aware what is going on.

Yesterday, when my son and a friend of his came, Carol asked Jim whether his wife has had her baby yet (It's due in 4 weeks). How frustrating it must be for her to know what is happening and not be able to communicate all of her thoughts.

A Month in the Hospital

Pray for our daughter, Robin, and our son Bob, that they make it here safely on Tuesday.

Love to all,
Bob

Received Monday February 26:

Bob,

Please know that we are praying for you and your family daily. We ask for continued guidance for you, as well as the peace that comes from knowing that God is in control and none of us is expected to have all the answers. Some things will only be answered when we are finally in His presence.

You and Carol have touched many lives. You are pillars in the Emmaus community, which is the only place that I've had contact with you. But I know that's only a small part of the work you do for the Lord. I specifically remember serving on Carol's walk in '95. I had the privilege of bringing her birthday cake for Sunday with the beautiful picture of our Shepherd with His sheep. What a comfort to know that our Shepherd is with us at all times, guiding us, loving us and holding us in His arms.

I pray that you, Carol, and your entire family can feel His arms around (and beneath) you right now. He knows your anguish and your confusion. He will undoubtedly lead you through this time of change.

Your Sister in Christ,
Trish Caldwell

Chapter 8

GOING HOME WITH HOSPICE

On Monday February 26 Bob wrote:

> Carol is coming home from the hospital on Wednesday morning under the care of hospice. They're delivering a hospital bed with a special mattress, oxygen, and everything we need to keep her comfortable. Yesterday they took out her feeding tube and with her stroke, she won't be able to swallow properly so we need your prayers that she won't have any discomfort here at home.
>
> Hospice nurses will come in a few times a week to check on her, but I'll be her main care-giver so I need your prayers also.
>
> Our two kids are coming from Phoenix and southern Indiana to help with her transition from hospital to home.

Dying with Carol

> Thank you again for
> your prayers,
> Bob

Received February 26:

Dear Bob,

I realize that it has been a long time since we've seen or spoken to each other, and I regret that it is under such painful circumstances that I am finally breaking my silence. Mom e-mailed me today regarding Carol's condition, and until I spoke with her last night, I had been unaware of Carol's illness. I just want you to know that I have thought of you and Carol and your family many times over the years despite the distance and the loss of contact, and I have nothing but fond memories of you all.

I also want you to know that I am praying for you all, especially that the Lord might give you the strength needed in the days ahead, and that you and Carol and the rest of your family might know the peace that only our Lord Jesus can give.

> Praying fervently, In Him,
> Bill Graack, Jr.

Bob wrote February 27:

We're bringing Carol home tomorrow under the care of hospice. We have a hospital bed set up in our living room

Going Home with Hospice

with a special air mattress and oxygen set up for her. Our two kids came in today and where Carol was thrilled to see them, I think, she also figured out the reason for both of them being here.

She also understands what hospice is. Our daughter Robin is staying with her tonight so I can sleep in our own bed and then tomorrow at 9:00 A.M., we will bring her home.

I'm not sure how long she will last because she won't be getting any nourishment. She can't swallow any food because of her stroke condition. She is not in any pain and I pray that she goes to Jesus before that starts.

Her brother, Cletus, and his wife Marty were coming in from New Mexico next Tuesday, but I called him and told him I couldn't promise she would still be with us by then.

I'm praying now that my lovely wife will be with the Lord as soon as he wills it.

Bob

Received February 27:

Dear Bob,

Thanks for the update. I am always glad to get them. Jim and I are holding you in our prayers.

Love Ya!
Marj

Dying with Carol

Dear Bob,

I pray that the Lord give you the strength and the courage to carry on once Carol is at home. We know that God will take her when He is ready and not a moment before. Be sure that you and the children tell her you will be fine, that she doesn't need to worry about you and then I know that you have released her to the Lord. My father had a stroke, after which he could not swallow, and he was on IV fluids only. I can't say that I know what you're going through because I don't, but I do know the good and faithful Father keeps His promises and we cling to them. When He says I will never leave you or forsake you, He means it. I pray that you and your family will feel His special touch as you care for Carol.

In His name,
Nancy Graf

Also received February 27:

You and Carol both continue to be in my prayers. Love you both so much.

Dalene

Home from the hospital.

On February 28 with the help of Methodist hospice, we moved Carol to our home in Eureka, Illinois. Our daughter Robin rode home with her in the ambulance and when we arrived, hospice had provided an air bed for Carol along with oxygen and a vacuum machine so that we could drain the fluid that was accumulating in her throat.

Going Home with Hospice

Bob wrote February 28:

> Carol is home and hospice is really amazing. They provided a hospital bed, with a special air mattress, oxygen, a vacuum to help drain the phlegm from her throat, all kinds of medication and training for me to take care of Carol.
>
> Our son Bob is going to stay with Carol while Robin and I go to Ash Wednesday services tonight.
>
> The out-pouring of love for us is really overwhelming. Cindy Grgurich, an old friend, came up from Decatur to see her this afternoon. We don't know how much longer we will have Carol with us, but with the help of hospice, we hope to keep her comfortable and free from pain.
>
> God bless you all,
> Bob

E-mails received February 28:

> Dear Bob and family,
>
> Please know my love and prayers are with you. It is so good to know where Carol will be, but oh I will miss her. She and you both were so helpful to me when I first started in prison ministry. May our God and loving Savior be so very real to your family at this time. May he wrap you in the arms of his tender love, even as he greets your beloved Carol. Tell her to tell Art, hello for me. (Art was her husband who was killed.) Every time a

Dying with Carol

friend goes home, I think that is one more who is waiting to greet us when we go home.

Love and prayers,
Violet

Bob,

Thinking and praying for you Carol and your family today as you bring her home from the hospital. If there is anything I can do for you, just let me know. This is a time for you as a family to spend time together. I'm so glad that you have your son & daughter there for support. We will be praying that the Lord spare Carol any pain.

We know your faith in the Lord will get you through this very difficult time. May God bless you and keep you in the days to come.

Your friends in Christ.
Linnie & Gary

My Precious Friend Carol,

Welcome home! You are surrounded in love and can lean back and rest in the arms of your loving Father.
In Jesus,

Chris

Dear Bob, Robin & Bob,

You may not read this until after I stop by, but I want you to know that I will be in Eureka today for a dental

Going Home with Hospice

appt. and lunch. I will stop by after lunch and if there is anything I can do, please let me know. I can fix a meal, answer the phone, clean the bathrooms, anything that would take a load off of the family. Please consider this and make a list for me.

Love,
Cindy

Chapter 9
49 DAYS WITH HOSPICE

On March 1 Bob wrote:

Late e-mail tonight

Last night our son Bob slept on the sofa next to Carol and about 2:15 A.M., I heard Carol coughing and then the throat vacuum going, so I knew Bob was trying to get the phylum from his mother's throat. I went down to our living room and for about an hour, we tried to make Carol comfortable. She finally went to sleep and her coughing stopped. She slept on and off today.

Her friend, Carolyn Shoof, stopped by with some miniature jonquils and Carol really smiled when she saw them. She is quite the flower lover and yellow is her favorite color.

Tomorrow the nurse will come again from hospice and also a nurse's aide to give her a bath. I'm praying that

Dying with Carol

she holds out until her brother Clete gets here from New Mexico.

Hospice gave us a book to look for signs of her passing and they are all there.

Thank you again for your prayers. Our good friend, Sue Ewan, sent a note today and suggested that we pray, "Oh Lord, let me have peace." She suggested that you won't be praying for me, but with me, as we pray my prayer.

> Thank you,
> Bob

E-mails received March 1:

> Just knew you would appreciate the loving care of hospice. Glad you were able to go to the Ash Wed. service. At ours, Dr. Bias's sermon was "Preparing for the Journey." You all are preparing for Carol's journey. Peace be with you, as much as possible.
>
> Love,
> The Kassings

On February 27 Bob sent this e-mail to Dalene Kuebler, who used to be the associate pastor of our church:

> Dalene,
>
> Scott is going to be gone until next Tuesday. If Carol dies before then, could you do the service? Scott said it is all right. In any case, I'd want you there because I

know you knew her and love her. I couldn't stand to have a minister doing the service that didn't know her.

Bob

Her reply on March 1:

Dear Bob,

I would be honored to take part in Carol's service. I had to think (and pray) about it though, I've been having bouts of homesickness and wondered how emotional it might be gathering with so many precious friends to say good-bye to another precious friend. But God has been asking me to trust Him more, and I believe He is asking me to trust Him on this one too.

Thank you for the ways you and Carol have trusted Him throughout all this. You continue to be a witness and an inspiration to us.

Huck and I are planning to be gone Friday and Saturday for our anniversary. We will be checking in at home and the church while we are away, so please feel free to leave a message if you need to get a hold of me.

God bless you.

Dalene

Bob's March 2 e-mail:

Both the RN and the LPN were here today to check on Carol and help give her a bath. The RN said her lungs

Dying with Carol

actually sounded a little better, but of course, Carol is not eating anything at all so she will be steadily be getting weaker. Hospice has provided morphine, not so much for pain, but to help with her irregular breathing. Sometimes she will go almost a minute between breaths. She appears to be getting more frustrated with her inability to communicate.

Tomorrow Carol's brother expects to get here from New Mexico. I know she is looking forward to that.

Father Purcell, who was the Catholic priest here in Eureka and was on the Cursillo team when I was rector, called today as well as Danny Cox, our United Methodist pastor of 10 years ago. He is now in Decatur, Illinois.

We have always been ecumenical in asking for prayers. I also talked to Jacquinot Weisenbach in Seattle, Washington, who is an old friend. They had one of their buildings damaged by the earthquake.

Carol has received over 350 e-mail prayers to date.

Thanks to all,
Bob

March 2 e-mails received:

Peace, Bob, peace.

May the peace of Christ rest with you and upon you. In His name I pray,

Amen

Bruce

49 Days with Hospice

Bob,

We are praying Sue's prayer with you as well as continually holding you all close in our hearts.

Love,

           Rich & Margo

Saturday March 2 Bob wrote:

Late Saturday night

Carol's talking is getting less and less, but she is still able to communicate for those of us around her. One thing she can do is wink with either eye to respond to us telling her how much we love her.

Her brother Clete, and his wife Marty came in from New Mexico tonight and you could tell from her eyes how much she appreciated it. She slept all of last night with the help of some medicine and we hope she will again tonight.

One thing this whole ordeal has impressed upon me is that friends and family are the most valuable thing we have in this world. We are all part of the "Body of Christ" and that love will last far beyond this thing we call life.

I have no idea how long she will be with us. She isn't taking any nourishment so it won't be too long. I now pray that the angels she talks about seeing will take her gently.

I feel closer to God now than I ever have before in my life.

Dying with Carol

> In His love,
> Bob

E-mails received March 3:

Dear Bob,

Carl and I have been praying daily for you and Carol. The thrill of her seeing Jesus face to face and knowing it is so fantastic. God's grace is tremendous. Peace and angels stationed around your beloved are prayers of ours.

> Love in Christ,
> Carl and Carolyn

Dearest Bob and family,

I await your e-mails each day with my prayers for all of you. I sat by my mother 8 years ago during each minute of her last 6 days. She was an angel on earth, like your beautiful Carol. They know what waits for them is grander than anything we can ever imagine on earth. I held my mother's hand and stroked her face at her last breath. She passed early on a Sunday morning as the sun rose. I miss her every second, but I know she's with me.

Bethany and I saw Carol 2 weeks ago on a Friday afternoon and I don't believe she knew us at that time. Please give her a kiss for us.

May God be with you though this difficult time.

> Our love and prayers,

49 Days with Hospice

Cindy, Don and Bethany

On March 5 Bob wrote:

The hospice nurse told us today that Carol's lungs were not as congested as they were five days ago. We realized this is because we haven't had to use the vacuum to clear her throat as often. Where this is good news, we have to remember that she is not taking any nourishment and very little water. Eventually Carol will become too weak to fight for those irregular breaths. We now know we are on God's time, so we must put everything in His hands.

Keep praying for us during
the struggle,
Bob

Received on March 5:

Bob,

I know the feeling of helplessness that you are feeling. I lost an Aunt to cancer two months ago and this sounds just like the way that she was. Her spirits were up all the way to the end and she went to be with our Father in her sleep. I wanted to tell you this before but I felt that the time wasn't right. I pray that when He calls her home that it will be at a time of no discomfort to her and a time of thanksgiving to your family knowing that she is with the one that matters the most!

Bob, you two have been and will always be an inspiration to Ann's and my walk with our Lord. You guys have

Dying with Carol

touched us and have helped nurture us to know our savior and God in ways that you will never know.

Ron Hursey

On March 6 Bob wrote:

Not too much to report. Carol listened to music today. She really likes the "Glory and Praise" songs and then I played a Tennessee Ernie old time song, "Mansions Over The Hill Top." If you remember that song or if you've never heard it, it will touch you. Another one that brought tears to my eyes is, "Thank You" for giving to the Lord.

Her breathing is still irregular and the nurse couldn't understand it because her lungs sound clear. We're afraid fluid is pushing the lungs and causing the irregularity.

We are giving her as much water as she can get from a small sponge on a stick, but that's the only fluid she is getting.

I'm going to sleep on the sofa next to her tonight and give my daughter, Robin, a break.

On a religious radio station today, I heard a minister say, "The more a good person suffers, the greater the reward in Heaven."

I don't know if that is true, but it may explain why Carol has had to go through all she has gone through since last September: breast cancer, ovarian cancer, a block bowel, a colostomy, and a stroke.

49 Days with Hospice

I know now God is preparing a mansion for her.

Love to all,
Bob

E-mails received March 6:

Dear Bob,

I am sorry that Carol has had to suffer so much. I am glad that you can still share music that you love. Jim, Jen and I are all praying for you throughout the days and nights.

Love ya!
Marj

Remember my Dear Brother in Christ,

That Carol is not suffering from not drinking. I have really been praying for you in this area tonight cause I have been on both sides as a care giver and one who took care of others.

It really bothers YOU when they do not eat or drink, but it does not bother Carol at all, her body is shutting down but that does not lessen the pain for the care givers who are watching and caring for her. My friend, who I am staying with here in Baltimore, asks about you daily. We both remember you in our prayers. See, there are people you have never seen that care and pray, pray and pray some more.

Dying with Carol

I am thankful you keep us all posted. I go to my e-mail several times a day to see if you or your kids have posted anything.

I pray this night, Oh Father God, as Bob lays on the couch by his dear wife for so many years, may You hold them together in your arms that they will feel an even more special bond than just husband and wife May they feel ONE in YOU.

Abba, care for the children and grandchildren. This is hard as you know, may they remember that life in you one day brings a close to this life and an opening of life eternal.

Abba, you know the needs of each one. I ask that you fill those needs and I ask this in your Son Jesus Christ's name.

Your sister in Christ
Julie Sechrest

Bob wrote Wednesday March 7:

Today a few friends came from church to see Carol and they were surprised she knew them. Carol does know what is going on. She only has a hard time expressing herself. She told Robin today she saw the Angel of Death. I think sometimes she is seeing things which we can't and yet she is still all with us.

We had to redo her colostomy today, but it came out all right. We are increasing some of her medication on the advice of the hospice nurse.

I don't know how long our daughter Robin can stay. She is a real "God-send." We're taking one day at a time.

Carol's brother, Clete and his wife, Marty are here with us every day.

I know all of the prayers are being heard by God. What we want now is that, "His will to be done."

Love to all,
Bob

Received March 7:

Hang in there, Bob, Robin & Bobby. You honor God in the way that you serve!

Blessings in Jesus.

John & Sue

This next e-mail was written by a high school classmate of Carol's and I lived in their house when I was working my way through college.

Dear Bob, Carol, and your whole family.

You are on my mind all the time and in my prayers. I still want you to heal and be back to good health again. I keep praying for the impossible, I guess, but I can't help it because this is really what we all want.

Dying with Carol

Carol–I keep thinking about you as I am fast walking my three miles around Seward Park (in the state of Washington) every morning thinking–here I am in great health, able to walk and be part of our wonderful nature, and you are my age lying in bed not able to do the same. It is so hard for me to absorb this. Seems just yesterday we were all together laughing at past events at the class reunion. I am wondering what it is like to see the Angels around you. We all wish we could witness this with you. Bob and I watch the TV program "Touched By An Angel" on Sunday nights and are often moved by the events.

If only . . . My Dear, Dear friend Carol . . . I wish I could once again be there to visit and to enjoy your many talents of china painting, quilt making, gardening with all your new plants, roses, bulbs . . . and so much more. You are a very special person loved by so very many who know you. I am wondering what your next journey will be . . . none of us get to know what our next adventure will be and who we will get to know during this time period. I can't help but wonder how many of us knew each other in another life and another time period. Just know that we will all be wondering how you are doing.

Bob, you knew my Dad . . . I still miss him terribly . . . and often "talk to him" He had such a presence! When I hiked down in the Grand Canyon for a week back in 1971, it seemed as though he was with me a lot.

This was just a year after he died. My Grandmother Amy died while I was down in the Canyon and no one was able to get a hold of me at the time so I was not able to be home for her funeral. As a result, I keep thinking that she's still here. It is really rotten when we lose our wonderful loved ones. I am so glad you got to know Mom and Dad those years you lived out at Collinwood with us.

Bob, I really do appreciate your keeping in touch with me and letting me know how Carol is doing. Thank goodness Clete was able to be with Carol too. I haven't seen Clete in years–tell him hello.

Once again I will close and send to all of you our love and prayers.

Tell Carol I love her.

Jacquinot and Bob

Also received March 7:

Hi Bob,

There has to be some reason Carol is hanging on. Sorry, but I still pray for a miracle.

I am sorry you and her kids have to go through this but it sure makes them realize how much they love Carol and you.

We went to a funeral today of a friend from church who was 87.

The funeral was really a celebration. He was a special gentleman.

Dying with Carol

You are in our prayers and on our hearts.

I have to go to Jacksonville tomorrow and pick up my blind grandson and take him home and stay until his folks get home from Mississippi.

Hopefully, I won't have to go through a lot of snow. Keep me posted. Life goes on. You need to take care of yourself.

Get out once in awhile. You need to.

Love you lots,
Marilyn

Received March 8:

Bob,

It must be tough to keep us all updated each day, but I look for the update first thing every morning and am able to align my prayers with what is in the update. If it gets too much for you to keep us informed, we will all understand, but hopefully you will be able to continue your daily reports.

My prayer is for peace in your home, no pain for Carol, peace in her mind when she wants to communicate and can't, and strength to continue the journey you are all on. My only real contact with you and Carol, once again, has been thru Emmaus, where I've always seen both of you as pure examples of Jesus in the flesh. Whether you know it or not, what you are going thru right now, and the fact that you take the time to share it with all of us, is probably your biggest act of "Jesus in the flesh."

You are ministering to so many of us with your example of faith, strength, love and everything good from God.

Bob, I wish I could give you and Dr. Carol (Ph D of Hugology) a great big HUG from me! And until I can, please know that my prayers are focused very heavily on all of you at this time.

Your Sister in Christ,
Trish Caldwell

Bob wrote on Thursday March 8:

So many people have responded that they read these messages daily and I am truly grateful for those of you who are sharing this time with us. Sometimes I wonder what I am going to say on a day when things take place just like so many days before.

Today we got out some of our old home movies (now on video) and Carol watched for a while before she went back to sleep. There we were a lot younger, full of life, and raising babies. God has blessed us in so many ways. He has used us and He has blessed us.

We received an e-mail from Trish Caldwell, who remembered Carol has the "Hug Doctor," a skit we used to do for women's Walks. The Lord used Carol and I in many ways and we are truly grateful.

Now I see her as vulnerable as a person can be. Her only request these days is for water. I thought of the sponge that was given our Lord on the cross and I imagine He appreciated it as much as Carol appreciates this simple act.

Dying with Carol

Thank God she is not experiencing any physical pain, but the lack of being able to speak clearly from her stroke does frustrate her.

Our son, Bob is coming back tomorrow with his wife, Jennifer, and we and Carol are looking forward to that. I don't know how long Carol will hold out. I guess her body can hold out for many days without food and very little water. We have told her it is all right to go, but her body is still struggling.

As I said last night, we are on God's time.

Bob

E-mail received March 9:

Bob—what a wonderful idea to share the movies with Carol. That allows her to review her life, even when she cannot speak. Many people review during their last few days, and you have made that possible for Carol and for you, too.

Continuing to lift you in prayer.

Blessings.

John & Sue

From some new Emmaus friends:

Dear Bob,

We would like to say that, through Sue, we seem to have a connection with both of you. Sue has often spoken of

Carol and the Reunion Group they shared. You have both been and are in our prayers and the prayers of many in our church, but more personally for us because of our close connection with Sue & John. We know how special you are to them.

While we can't fully appreciate your struggles and pain, we do understand the joy of a life lived together for so many years. We will continue to pray for strength for you, Bob and for peace for Carol. Each day we will carry you both softly in our hearts and lift you gently in our prayers.

In Christ's love
Louise & Duane

Bob,

I for one am honored and grateful that you let me share in a very emotional and personal time. My heart reaches out to you and your family each day. I check for your messages each day to see how you and Carol are doing. It helps me to hear how you are feeling that day because it gives me a direction to go with my prayers for you. I am in awe of your closeness and faith in God in what is undoubtedly the most painful and trying time in your life. I can only hope and pray that I would be as strong as you in a similar situation. I will continue to pray for you all.

Your sister in Christ,
Cherie Barr

Dying with Carol

Bob wrote on Friday March 9:

It's hard to imagine how many people love us until something like Carol's affliction takes over. This morning my secretary of fifteen years ago drove 16 miles to deliver some home made muffins to us. She didn't come in to see Carol because she was still sleeping. We had four different floral arrangements brought today. I am overwhelmed by the out-pouring of love and concern that has come from our friends around the state.

We're waiting for our son and his wife to come up from southern Indiana tonight.

An old friend, Krista Brockman, who will be ordained an elder in the United Methodist Church in June, came by tonight and was talking to Carol about the new body she could look forward to.

Another old friend, Marj Crowe, who sponsored Carol and I to Cursillo in 1977 was here today. After she left, I thought about all of the people who may have been indirectly touched by the simple act of asking her "principal" to make a Cursillo. Marj was a special education teacher for me back then and I have always said, "One way to straighten out a public school is to have the principal make a Cursillo or Walk to Emmaus."

Carol and I are just simple people. We aren't rich in material things, but throughout all of Carol's health problems, I can really see that we are the most blessed people on the face of the earth.

God bless you all,
Bob

49 Days with Hospice

E-mail received March 10:

> I had no idea things had gotten so bad with Carol until I talked to Cindy Shuford yesterday at work. She has forwarded me your e-mails of the last ten days or so. I am so sad for you yet happy at the same time. What love you have for your wife. I am deeply moved. I used to work at the beauty shop almost twenty years ago where Carol got her hair done. She became an instant friend. Time went by of course, and I started a family and would see Carol once a year even though we lived right here. Bruce and I started coming to your church (I have since gone back to my roots in the Catholic church), but oh how happy I was to see my old friend Carol standing at the entrance.
>
> When you talked about her being the "hug doctor," you couldn't have given her a more accurate title. She greeted me every Sunday, whether we were at the early or late service. She was there to give hugs to all at BOTH services. Her embrace is that of a loving, God sharing person. I love her.
>
> We had an opportunity to talk at the Chanticleer before her breast surgery and shared some thoughts on Dr. Jalovic. I trust she did her best for you, as I thought she was a wonderful doctor.
>
> Like I said, I had no idea Carol had gotten so ill and gone through all of these things since not coming to Methodist anymore. Please know and share with Carol that I am praying for her and all of your family. The care

Dying with Carol

and love you are giving her is coming from the Lord himself. What a tribute to Him and to Carol.

If she can understand, tell her I am thinking of her and love her and appreciate all the love she has given me.

God's Blessings,
JoEtta Hinrichsen

Bob sent this e-mail March 10:

Our son Bob came in last night with his wife Jennifer. He plans to stay for a while, but Jennifer will go back to Greenville, Indiana tomorrow.

It is good to have he and Robin here. Carol really thrives when they are around. It's been 12 days since Carol had any nourishment. She still is taking water by the sponge, but that is all. Hospice told us that she would not want any food and they were right. She is starting to see things the rest of us can't see. I think there are times now when she appears to be sleeping with her eyes wide open.

We are still being overwhelmed by the love of our friends. When I first started writing these e-mail messages, I felt that maybe I was placing my burden on others, and I probably am, but Carol and I have always been very open people and have shared our joys and our sorrows with others.

For those of you in a Cursillo or Emmaus reunion group, you know what I mean. Perhaps this is what I am doing now, except the reunion group has expanded to our many Christian friends and family.

Let us all pray together that Carol will let go of whatever is holding her to life and move to the new glory that will be hers in Jesus Christ our Lord.

Bob

E-mails received March 10:

Hi Bob

You and Carol remain daily in our prayers at this time. I think of all the ways the two of you have touched our lives directly and how that 'touching' impacts all those we are constantly in contact with. Each time I read your mail I am impressed with the thought that God is not through with the two of you yet. You continue to bring Him glory until the day that you each face Him face to face. Isn't that an awesome thought. We love you both.

Carl & Carolyn Wiggins

Dear Bob,

When our friend and mentor, Deacon Bill Fry, was at the end of his life here on earth, he prepared his family for his leaving. One of the beliefs he had was that he would slip from time to time "through the veil" separating this world from the next. Then he would slip back. He told them that there would come a time that he would go through the veil one last time and not return. His family tells me that this is exactly what happened.

One afternoon he went gently through the veil. He did not return to his old body. However, I can assure you from my own past experiences, he is still very near. I

Dying with Carol

just said recently that his wife of 50 years sounds more like him in the past five than I would have ever thought possible. He is still there whispering to her and to Jim and I.

I am learning about Celtic Spirituality. I find the concept of "thin places" very interesting. That has to do with those places or persons where the distance between the natural and the supernatural is very "thin."
Perhaps that is where Carol is when she sees things that others do not.

My prayers for all of you continue as you care for Carol so lovingly.

Thanks for being willing to share this part of your journey with those of us who love you.

Love Ya!
Marj

Other March 10 e-mails:

Bob,

Please do not feel you are a burden or that you are just "dumping" your problems on others. If someone doesn't want to read about your wife's "progress" towards a new life, all they need do is delete the message. On the other hand, I for one read with great interest every e-mail you send. I am curious about how you, Carol, and your family handle and cope with this time of spiritual struggle and grief.

It is my prayer that God will bless you richly. I remember a passage of Scripture where Jesus says, "I give you peace. Not the peace of this world but my peace." I pray that you receive that peace in the blessed name of Jesus.

Brother Clayton

Dear Bob,

Jacquinot phoned with a message about Carol. I am so sad and want you to know that my prayers are with you and your family. I had sent you an e-mail earlier but I didn't have the address right. I hope this reaches you.

Virginia Knowles
an EHS classmate of
Carol's in Prescott, Arizona

Bob wrote Sunday March 11:

Yesterday two old Emmaus friends, Linda Meachum, and Dottie Nickles, drove all the way from Champaign to visit with Carol for a few minutes. One of the things we find out from our Cursillo Emmaus experience is different acts of agape love. That is an example of the undeserved love of God. The number of e-mail responses is another example of this. In Cursillo we call it "palanca."

I have the feeling that God is using Carol's illness as a way for all of us to show what true Christian love is really like.

Dying with Carol

This morning in church our praise band played "I'll Fly Away." Where it is a joyful song, I found tears rolling down my cheeks because Carol and I both remember our 6 year old son singing that with such enthusiasm. The words "When I die, Hallelujah, By and By, I'll fly away" also brought tears.

I don't know why God is waiting to take Carol home. I know I will miss her terribly, but seeing her in the state where she can't express herself completely and although, not in pain, she is uncomfortable much of the time.

Krista Brockman was here a few days ago and was telling Carol of the new glorious body she will have. For a person like Carol who was so full of life to be bed-ridden and helpless, it must be frustrating.

I know that God is in control of this situation. Carol always told me I lack patience. God is reminding me that his time is not our time.

Thank you all again for all your expressions of agape love for both of us.

Bob

E-mails received March 12:

Dear Ones,

The song "I'll Fly Away" really struck me this morning in worship. As a teacher, I try to get my students to "feel" the words written by others. Close your eyes for a moment and "feel" the words "I'll fly away–OH, GLORY– I'll fly away." Whisper those words and imagine yourself unencumbered by your earthly body and "flying away" into the open arms of a beaming Jesus.

What joy we can all look forward to on that day.

In His love,
Chris

Hi Bob,

Kathern here again, I hope you don't mind my little messages I send. You seem to be in better spirits, as best that can be under the circumstances.

At the Emmaus closing last night we lifted you, Carol and your family up in prayers of the people. Sometimes trusting God is so hard to do, we stand on the promises in his Word, we pray, we be still to rest and listen, and yet nothing seems to come. I'm sure you have cried out "where are you God"? I have over the past three months. He seems to just be silent. The other day I was talking to God, if I could only see beyond today, what is going to happen, so I would at least know. Then God in his very gentle voice reminded me that if he showed me beyond today, there would be no reason to trust him.

Just as Rahab waited to be delivered for seven days while they marched around Jericho, we too have to wait, trusting God, that he does love us, he does have a plan and we sometimes can't see what or why he is doing but we know that all things work for good to those who love him.

If nothing else, God has shown you Jesus in the flesh and that his grace should be sufficient for us. I will keep praying for you daily, and just as God loves you, so do I. Just keep renewing your strength from the Lord, in his time he will give us the answers and show us what it is we are to see from all of this.

Love and prayers,
Kathern

Another e-mail:

Again, Dear friend, I want to say you have my love and prayers. We prayed again in church for you yesterday, as we always do. Pastor Dennis remembers you as a good coach and leader. He said, "Bob is just so real." I said amen. He and Carol both are.

Give Carol my love,
Violet

Another March 12 e-mail:

Bob:

Please don't stop sending them to me. I love you both and each one is a call to prayer for me on your behalf. I wish I could get there to hug you both, but I doubt that will happen.

Please know that I love you and my heart aches for both of you. I, too, have prayed for God to be merciful to Carol. And to you, too.

Bruce

49 Days with Hospice

Dear Bob,

I know this is probably therapy for you to write to us each day, but it is so thoughtful, too. I feel that I am a part of all your trials and glories! It blesses my day to hear from you and know that my prayers are focused to what you want for Carol.

Thanks for letting all of us be with you at this time. It means so much for us, too.

I have a request for you both–I am to be the Lay Director for the women's Walk in May. How I would have loved to have Carol on my team, but just remember how much she has meant to so many on other teams. I am asking that you be prayer warriors for my team. Pray with Carol that we have God's true choices in mind. I would be so blessed if you could do this–am I asking too much? I know that both of you have a direct line to Him–and would consider it one last task that Carol can do–to pray with you for those to be called–or have been called. Maybe this is one of those prayers that will help her let go–to know the wonderful love she has passed on and take it to our Creator in person.

I love you both and thank you for being such a bright light for Christ in my life.

Love,
Judy McKinney

Dying with Carol

Bob, you dear thing,

You certainly should not stop sending the e-mails. I check two or three times a day specifically to see if you have sent an update. I appreciate so much being informed. I love you and want to know how to pray for you.

Love to you and your family,
Chris

Bob,

We really appreciate getting your daily letters, as we can keep updated on our prayers for Carol, you and your children. Our thoughts and prayers are with you all every day. Our love to all of you.

Your friends in Christ,
Larry and Ruth Roach

Other March 12 e-mails:

Dear Bob,

I have come to know you and Carol from the time she gave out the hand encouragement notes for the Walk she was supposed to be on. I also suppose that praying for someone for a length of time is God's way of making them friends in one's heart. I know that at the times I have e-mailed you, you probably haven't had a clue who I am, and that is OK but I certainly appreciate the updates you send daily. They help me know how to pray;

when I wanted to stop praying for physical healing and start praying for comfort and strength for you and your family and peace for Carol. I wish I had known her, she must be quite a lady. My love to you and your family in Christ.

Nancy Graf

Dear Bob

My name is Darlene Wood and my husband John was on a Cursillo weekend with you back in September of 1999. Even though we have never met, I feel that I have come to know you and your family quite well through your e-mail messages. I so admire your strong faith and courage through this ordeal. Thank you so much for sharing your feelings and faith with us. We are keeping your whole family in our prayers.

Dear Bob,

Although I haven't taken time to write to you until now, we have been praying for you daily. We pray each and every day for you to be surrounded by angels.

And also for the Lord to take good care of you and Carol. As for your last statement about stopping the e-mails: DON'T YOU DARE STOP. Also they are a good reminder to pray, (just in case I get so wrapped up in my own affairs).

Dying with Carol

We love you both. God Bless You.

Harold & Carolyn Turner

The last of the March 12 e-mails:

Hello Bob

Sorry I haven't been able to be in touch the past two nights. Bob has been busy on this computer with so many things that I haven't been able to do my own thing. Thank you so much for the updates—I feel that we are with you every step of the path that you and Carol are taking on this long and very upsetting journey. My heart goes out to all of you.

Watching your loved one slowly leaving this earth must be wrenching. I feel blessed every day to be healthy and able. I am so glad that you have many wonderful friends that are there helping you, and so many from the church.

Virginia Karl Knowles called me Sat. night to find out how Carol was doing. I had called her some time back and gave the news about the blockage and the terrible condition Carol was facing. She had been gone for a couple of weeks. I see by your e-mail addresses that she is now on your list too, so she managed to be in touch from your e-mail that I gave her. I don't know if you remember that she had a bout with breast cancer a couple of years ago.

I can't imagine how Carol is surviving all this torture. We are both praying for both of you. Please, do keep your e-mails coming!

49 Days with Hospice

Love,
Bob and Jacquinot

Bob wrote Sunday March 12:

Things got somewhat worse for Carol today because she started to vomit from time to time. How anyone could, who hasn't had a bite of food for 13 days really makes you wonder. The hospice nurse, after conferring with our doctor, thinks the cancer has caused another bowel blockage. We don't want to take her back to the hospital and have a tube put into her stomach so we're going to try to control the nausea with medication. One of them a pill that costs $100.00 a day. Thank God hospice is paying for them. We're just trying to make her as comfortable as we can. The nurse is amazed that Carol still recognizes her every other day.

Sunday morning Carolyn Schoof, our church choir director, came between services and sang some of Carol's favorite hymns.

I don't know how I could have handled this without the help of our two kids. Carol and I have been really blessed in that regard.

I'm praying now that the Lord take her before she has any more discomfort.

Bob

Dying with Carol

E-mails received March 13:

Greetings Bob,

Know that you and Carol continue to be in my prayers. Know also that you are both loved by a lot of people. I wish I could be there to give you a hug, so check the floor and then consider yourself hugged.

God Bless,
Pastor John M. Cross
Sadorus/Parkville UMC

(John is a big man as am I. He made his Emmaus when I was lay leader. After that experience he went into the ministry; we also joked that they had to reinforce the floor when we stood together and hugged.)

Don't take ME off your e-mailing list. Yours is the FIRST one I open each morning. I even check near the end of my workday to see if you've slipped in an extra one. Your words are a ministry in and of themselves and I feel truly blessed by your allowing me to share with you at this time.

Our prayers continue to be with you all.

Trish Caldwell

Keep 'em coming and thank you for your sharing. Am sure your kids and community continue to be such a source of strength. How neat that a choir member came to sing some of Carol's favorite hymns.
God bless.

The Kassings

49 Days with Hospice

Hi Bob,

Glad that God has given you time to tell her that you love her.

Ann and I have only been married for 17 yrs. But when I say, "Ann, you know what?" She always comes back and says, "I know you love me" and with us smiling at each other I say, "You took the words right out of my mouth."

God's blessings on you both.

> Just trying to be his servant,
> Ron

Dear Bob and Carol,

I can't tell you how overwhelmed I was by your response to my note. You have so many friends and so many e-mails. I thank God too that He has given you the time to hold each other's hands, say I love you, and just "be" together.

What a beautiful picture that paints in the midst of the storm. Know that my love goes out to both of you as well as my prayers. I just completed team work on walk 147. The theme of the walk was Ps. 91:1–2. It seems appropriate for all of us and I know that you both dwell in the shadow of the most high. My prayer for you today is to thank God for the medication working and to praise him for knowing what is the best for both of you right now, as we humans couldn't possibly know.

In Jesus,
Nancy Graf

More e-mails received:

Dear Bob,

I have been reading your e-mails as you have kept all of us informed on Carol's condition. I was saddened to hear Carol's fight with cancer is nearing an end. Yet at the same time I know she will be rewarded greatly in heaven. That is our ultimate goal, to return to our father and have life eternal, yet there is always the side of us which grieves for our loss. It is saddest for those who may never have the chance to know her and serve with her in advancing God's Kingdom here on earth. She will always live in our hearts, a part of her is always within each of us. It is a great sacrifice to care for a loved one, but it is a precious time you have. I pray for all of you during this time. May God continue to comfort you and lift you up, give you all strength to endure.

I wish I could come see you both. Tell Carol I'm thinking of her. She probably won't be able to recognize who you are talking about, but that's okay. Just know you are in my thoughts and prayers. I have not seen you guys in quite some time. I have sort a of retreated from a lot in the last 3 1/2 years, just trying to survive the pain of an incident.

I will pray for all of you, and your hospice nurse too.

49 Days with Hospice

Bonnie Devore

Bob sent this e-mail Tuesday March 13:

Carol is still hanging in there. She still knows what is going on around her and she recognizes everyone. Her hospice nurse is really amazed as to her stamina. It's been 14 days now since she has had anything to eat. We have found the drug hospice gives us helps her nausea. So far that is under control.

I realize today that this period we're going through is giving us more quality time together than we have had in years. We've both been busy with church and our different ministries, but it is if God signaled a "Time Out," just so we could hold hands and tell each other of our love. I hate to admit it, but I have told my wife I love her more in the last 6 weeks than I probably have in the last six years.

Not that I didn't love her, but after 45 years, we men have a tendency to expect our wives to know it.

If there are any husbands reading this, will you tell your wife you love her for me tonight?

Love to all,
Bob

E-mail received:

Bob,

I'm sorry I haven't been able to get over to see you and Carol or do anything for you and your family. We are praying for all of you. We know this is difficult for all of you. We look forward to your updates on Carol.

Last night we were sitting on the couch watching TV and Gary looked over and said I love you. I said what brought that on. He said in your e-mail that all men getting this message tell your wife you love her. In all the pain you are going through you are still ministering to those of us receiving your e-mails. Gary and I are leaving for Florida Sat. and returning on March 31. Marilyn is going to keep us updated on Carol's condition. We will be praying for all of you even though we are not here. Just know God is in control. In all things His will be done. Love to all of you.

Gary & Linnie

Bob,

My sister-in-law has been forwarding me your e-mail messages almost every single day. I have followed Carol's illness and have prayed for you and Carol throughout.

At church the week before last, I prayed especially for Carol to be comforted by angels, and that evening was when you sent out an e-mail saying Carol was seeing angels and I was so happy for her.

My heart goes out to you all . . . know that I'm praying for and loving you both . . .

Sherry Howard
Lebanon, KY

49 Days with Hospice

Bob wrote Tuesday March 15:

> Our kids had to make a hard decision today, but they have family responsibilities of their own. The hospice chaplain told me, "There is no wrong decision under these circumstances."
>
> Tomorrow, our son Bob is renting a car to go back to Louisville and he's taking our daughter, Robin, to Indianapolis to catch a Southwest Airline back to Phoenix.
>
> I won't be alone, however, because Carol's brother and his wife, who have been staying at other people's houses will come and stay here.
>
> We're helping Carol to sleep more and more because of her intestinal problems bother so much when she's awake.
>
> The days are running together so much I have to remind myself of what day it is. Today is rainy and dreary and it doesn't help the sad mood around here.
>
> An old friend, Jim Behme called today. He used to be the lay leader of the Peoria Cursillo. Also, some friends from the Roanoke Benson Junior High where I last served as principal stopped by.
>
> I wonder what the kids' leaving will do for Carol tomorrow. She understands, but our daughter, Robin knows she will probably will never see her mother alive again.
>
> Please say a special prayer for her.

Dying with Carol

Love to all,
Bob

E-mails received Thursday March 15:

Bob,

I don't really know what to make of Carol's hanging in there, but I think it is awesome, the love of your family that she gets from you and your children. I have never thought of death as a beautiful experience, but I have heard people call it that. Even though I am not there, the love that I feel emanating from you for your wife bleeds through your e-mails. I am deeply moved.

Please know that my thoughts and prayers are with you. Carol is truly a blessing. Love to all of you and if she can understand, please tell her I love her. She's a great lady and I am praying for her.

JoEtta

Bob, I just read your e-mail about the kids leaving. I know exactly how they feel, especially Robin. Give her a hug for me. Also, call me if I can be of assistance.

Love,
Iris

Bob,

You are just facing very challenging times–many decisions for many people, especially your kids. Know

49 Days with Hospice

Robin's decision must be gut-wrenching. They came to serve and to say good bye.

Prayers continue.

Love,
The Kassings

Dear Bob,

Thursday evening I attended UMW at church. Cindy Shuford shared with me the e-mail she had received from you about your children having to return to their homes. I just want to let you know that all of you are in my thoughts and prayers. Carol and you are special people in my life.

Joyce Borzello

Bob wrote on Friday March 16:

In many ways, Carol is recovering from the stroke. She can take water from a straw now and is speaking more distinctly, but her bowel blockage is keeping her from any food or desire for food.

The hospice nurse said today that her blood pressure was up which might indicate pressure building up in her brain and the possibility of another stroke. She took her blood pressure just an hour after Robin and Bob left so that may have caused that reaction.

Dying with Carol

It is amazing how strong Carol still is without any kind of nourishment for 17 days now. The nurse says it's unbelievable.

I know Carol is far better off in our home with us taking care of her than in a hospital or a nursing home.
Carol's brother, Clete and his wife Marty moved in to help me out today.

Carol seems to accept the kids leaving all right, but when I stepped out of the room to tell them good-bye, when I came back in the room she had a scared look in her eye and said very clearly, "You're not leaving!" I assured her I would never leave her.

Last night she asked if she would ever be able to paint again.

For those of you who have never been to our house, it is filled with hand painted china that Carol has done over the years. When Robin and I talked about that later on the phone, we decided that if she did it would be in heaven.

Thanks again for
your prayers,
Bob

E-mail received March 16:

Dear Bob

I am sure there have been very difficult decisions for you and the kids to make. I will pray for safety for Bob and Robin as they travel, and also for God's peace to fill their hearts and yours.

The first part of the week we attended a clergy conference in Peoria. Krista was several rows over from me, but during one of the worship times I could hear her voice loud and clear over all the others around me. I told her later that that is how I will find her in heaven—I will recognize her voice. Carol will be right inside the gate greeting all who come through with a brightly colored robe, a big smile and a warm hug!

Josh still talks about you as being that big man who wasn't afraid to get up in front of the church and sing "Jesus Wants Me for a Sunbeam."

Thank you for being a witness not only to me, but to my family, and to all whose eyes are upon you now.

Dalene

Dearest Bob, Carol, and Family,

You are in my heart and prayers today as always. Let's keep trusting Jesus. It is Jesus who has the final say (not illness), and we know that what He has in store for you, Carol, is a perfectly beautiful life with Him. You are dearly loved, my precious friend.

In Him,
Chris

Dying with Carol

Bob wrote March 17:

Carol's main problem now seems to be nausea from her bowel blockage and being uncomfortable lying in her bed. She's been in bed since January 29 and even though she has a special bed it still is uncomfortable.

Just now as I left to go upstairs to our computer room, she warned me don't go too far. I don't know if she is trying to tell me something or even if she feels something herself. It's not as if she were alone. There were four people with her as I left.

I don't know if she is building resistance to some of the medicine, but it seems the effects wear off in a shorter time now. She is waking up now in the middle of the night. In the hospital sometimes she would sleep the night through.

Keep praying that God gives her rest and peace.

Love to all,
Bob

E-mail received March 17:

Bob and family

Thank you for keeping us informed of Carol and for sharing in this most precious yet difficult time. You have all been in my prayers daily. How frustrating it must be to see her discomfort and not be able to help her relieve that pain. I wish we understood God's plan for her. Please know that we think of you each day. Thank you for being brave enough to rely on your friends and family for help and prayers. Please give Carol a hug for me and be sure to do the same for yourself. Take care.

> Peace to you . . .
> Kelly

Dear Bob,

Jim e-mailed me about your wife and a special prayer for you and your wife. God Bless you and your family. Thoughts and prayers are with you always. Our deepest prayers are with you.

God Bless.

> Patrick Kelly

Bob wrote March 18:

> We're giving Carol more morphine now as her discomfort grows. Last night she complained how weak she feels and this morning early, she complained about being short of breath. Still that great heart of hers keeps beating and she is fully alert to what is going on. This morning as I was bringing her some fresh water, I spilled a little coming into the room and she told me that I did and I'd better wipe it up so it doesn't stain the carpet. That's my old Carol.
>
> It's even more important for me now to sleep on our sofa next to her because she gets anxious if I'm out of her sight too long. She did give me the OK to go to church

this morning. Her brother and his wife will stay with her Her nights have fallen into a pattern of sleeping until about 12:30 then when I give her the scheduled medication she stays awake for and hour until they kick in. Then she sleeps from about 1:30 A.M. to 5:30 A.M.

As I said before, she does know she is getting weaker. It's about 20 days now since she's had any nourishment.

Keep praying,
Bob

E-mails received March 18:

Hi Brother Bob;

I have been thinking about you and Carol since I got on line to get your messages. I continue to hold you and yours up in prayer to have the patience to wait on God to do His will. These lingering deaths are tough, as I remember from the death of my father several years ago.

But, as we know it is in God's time! I know the angels are around you and Carol and they are awaiting God's signal to come and get her for her eternal home. So we can pray and wait and reflect on the good times in God's presence over our years. So I pray and encourage you in this time of testing.

Thanks for your updates. Remember God loves you and I love you too!!!

Bye for now,
Paul

49 Days with Hospice

Another March 18 e-mail received:

> Our prayers are still with you Bob, for comfort for you and Carol and for peace for both of you and that you can feel the presence of our Lord in the room with you. Keep your eyes on what He might be doing during this time.
>
> Our love reaches out to both of you,
Nancy and Karl Graf

> I heard about your wife during the summer and this was unexpected news. I feel bad for not getting in contact with you then Bob. Thanks for your e-mail and by all means our prayers are with you and Carol (also your family). I believe God gives all of us second chances. Thoughts and prayers are with you both. God Bless. You are in our prayer chain.
>
> Patrick

Bob's March 19 e-mail:

> It will be three weeks since Carol has had any nourishment tomorrow. I thought we might lose her twice today. She complained about not being able to breath, but with the help of some medicine, her breathing was restored to semi-normal and she is still with us.
>
> The hospice nurse has given us permission to give her some of the medication at shorter time intervals so we may be able to keep her discomfort to a minimum.
>
> We had several visitors today. Some old friends we haven't seen in years and some loyal church friends.

Dying with Carol

If people come to visit us, I want them to know that if Carol is mercifully sleeping we aren't going to wake her. I am so grateful for the times when her eyes are closed and I know she has no pain or discomfort.

We are trying to control her nausea from her new bowel blockage. Right now, that is our main concern. I am positive she is aware that her time with us is limited. God only knows what his time schedule for Carol's time on earth is. I'm grateful for the times we still have together holding hands and looking into each other's eyes.

I am well aware that shortly; I will not have that.

Love to all.

Bob

E-mails received March 19:

Dear Bob,

Thank you for the putting me on your list. I returned to last week's messages and along with you am amazed at the strength Carol is displaying.

She is not ready to leave yet. Her strength is giving all of us a chance to become stronger and to prepare for the time when she won't be with us. My prayers are with you all.

Virginia

Bob,

John Ewan has kept me updated on Carol. Am praying for her and your family. I'm sorry I didn't stop when Robin was there.

Sending love and prayers.

Phyllis Troyer

Dear Bob,

It sounds like you are treasuring the moment to hold hands with Carol and look into those eyes of love.

Peace and rest to you,
The Kassings

P.S. Thank you for sharing with us.

Bob wrote March 20:

> Right before Carol fell asleep last night, she said to me, "I'll see you in heaven." She was still with me at 3:00 A.M. when I gave her some medication and she is still with us today. What this tells me is that her mind and her spirit are ready, but her body is still fighting to stay alive.
>
> She has lost so much weight, she probably weighs less now than when we were married forty-five years ago. She still is alert.
>
> This morning her brother was fixing some french toast and she recognized the smell and asked her brother to

save some for her. She doesn't eat anything which is a blessing because with her bowel blockage it would just come up and make her miserable.

We tried a little apple juice the other day, but she couldn't tolerate it.

According to the hospice book, even without a bowel blockage at this stage of dying, the body refuses food. Most of us, in our living process, never think about the death process. During the last seven weeks, God has given me a lot of time to learn about it. I guess all we can pray for now is that her body and her mind and spirit become attuned.

In His Love,
Bob

E-mails received March 20:

Dear Carol,

This e-mail is just for you, precious friend. I want you to be aware of something the Lord just prompted me to do. I scheduled days on my calendar for the rest of the year when I would be sure to pray for your family. I know how much you love your husband, children, grandchildren and your brother and his wife. You will be in the best place of all to discuss them with the Lord, but I know you also value the prayers of friends. Rest assured that your loved ones will be in mine, and I ask that you remember my family in yours as you always have. You have been a faithful, praying child of God, Carol. His arms are out to you now. You are dearly loved.

> In Him,
> Chris

Another March 20 e-mail:

> Certainly will be praying, Bob. Caring for dying people as a Stephen's Minister has been as experience for me and when my father died, it was really helpful to know kind of what to expect. My prayer for you is still peace and comfort and the strength to do the day-to-day things. What a blessing that you can hold her hand and talk to her and know she understands you.
>
> My love to both of you.
>
> > Nancy Graf

> Dear Bob, I give thanks for your strong faith. Getting your messages every day is a real witness to the strength that those who love the Lord can bear much. I am struck by how much better it is to know that your days are numbered. Compare this with the shock of losing someone in an accident. May your faith continue to sustain you.
>
> > Fondly,
> > Virginia

> Just a note to let you know I've been thinking of you. Tell Carol we all love her and miss her. She's a great lady. Our prayers are with you.
>
> > Love,
> > Diane and Al

Dying with Carol

Bob's e-mail; March 21:

> The battle to keep Carol comfortable from stomach nausea is becoming more difficult. The medicine we give her seems to work for three hours, but we can only give it to her every four hours. By using a suppository in the middle of the night (through her colostomy) I was able to let her sleep for a full 8 hours last night, but today when the C.N.A. came she didn't feel up to having a complete bath because of her nausea. I wonder what other damage the ovarian cancer is doing to her body.
>
> How she is living off her body reserves is really amazing. The last nourishment she had was February 27. She is still aware of her surroundings and still smiles when she sees a familiar face.
>
> The routine of this vigil is difficult for her brother, his wife, and me. Robin and son Bob call each day and all I can say is no change.
>
> Lord, give us the strength to support Carol and to determine her needs.
>
> Love to all.

March 21 e-mails received:

> Lifting you both to the Lord. Read Ps. 84:4–7 and know that strength.
>
> Blessings,
Sue

49 Days with Hospice

Bob wrote March 22:

> Everything goes on the same. Carol is getting more fearful because she knows she is getting weaker. Not fearful of death, but fearful that something will happen and she won't be able to respond. We must be with her at all times. Last night at 3:00 A.M. she wanted me to call the fire department. She dreamed our house was on fire and she couldn't escape it. It must be horrible to be fully aware of what is going on or dreaming and know that your body is too weak to respond and save you.
>
> She wants me with her most of the time. Today I had to make a trip to Peoria to get her some medicine. Luckily, her friend Jane was here with her brother and sister-in law.
>
> For those who knew Carol as a "full figured" woman, you wouldn't recognize her now. I do because she looks a lot like the Carol I married.
>
> Our kids don't know what to do. It's much harder on them than it is on me, because I am where I should be and there is no decision to make.
>
> Pray for our kids, Robin and Bob.
>
> Bob

E-mails received March 22:

> Hello Bob,
>
> Can't tell you how glad I am you are sending us the daily updates. I hope you and Carol know how much you both

mean to us and have over many years in our daily Christian walk. The first time we ever came to Eureka Methodist (Rev. Flynn did not use the "United" term at the time), I remember meeting Carol. Bobby was just a tiny little boy and he had become restless in church and Carol took him out. We were sitting in the back and I was feeling very shy and new but as Carol walked down the aisle with Bobby, she smiled at me. I will never forget it because it was such a warm, welcoming smile it made me think maybe this would be a church home for us.

That was just the beginning of many times God has worked through the two of you. We are all struggling to make some sense of Carol's pain and the difficult time you are all having. But God has used you and Carol so many times without you even knowing it; we have to continue to trust that He will continue to do so. Even through this. Just know that you are in our thoughts and prayers continuously.

Please tell Carol I love her.

Love,
Margo

Bob and family,

Just want you to know I'm still praying. Thanks for keeping us informed . . . God is still God and he is still using Carol to bless our lives. What a ministry even on her death bed and through your e-mails . . . our lives are touched. Blessed be the name of our Lord.

Love and prayers,
Violet

Another March 22 e-mail:

> You've got the prayers–know that this is not easy for anybody. Praying that your time together will be a blessing to you both as you come to appreciate this struggle for Carol's new birth into heaven. It is always harder on the baby as the birthing process begins, than during the 9 months.
>
> Keep holding her hand as you walk her home.
>
> Love to you both.
>
> Sue

Bob's March 23 e-mail:

> Carol had a good night. She slept through almost 8 hours. I was able to give her the medicine through a suppository at 2:00 A.M. without waking her up.
>
> Her nurse and the C.N.A. came about 4:00 P.M. and replaced a lot of her medication ports etc. It really wore her out, but at least now she is through that for another week.
>
> We have families from our church bringing in meals three times a week and we really appreciate it.
>
> We have been able to decrease the times between some of Carol's medications which seem to help. It's hard for me to believe how much weight she has lost and how little flesh she has left on her bones. When she is awake we struggle to get her into a comfortable position. It

may mean adjusting pillows and her position every few minutes.

I know there are many people praying for her and us. I know God's plans will work out. Give us the patience to see it through.

Love to all,
Bob

March 23 e-mails received:

It is really good that you are able to share this time. Love to you both.

John & Sue

Hi Bob,

I am thinking of you—hoping you and Carol can see a beautiful sunshiny day outside your window. The daffodils are coming up and the pussy willows are about to burst open. I enjoy my drive across the lake each day, because in March beautiful seagulls come from the south and just cover the lake.

I think it is such a great sight to see them soaring above the water. Too soon they will move on to the north, perhaps Lake Michigan and beyond to cool nights and warm days.

I am just about to finish calling my team together; thank you for your prayers! I'm sure you are praying for the team and pilgrims meeting at Dwight in another week.

How I miss going up there. After I'm put out to pasture on the street Walks, then I can go to the prisons again.

Judi Robbins cannot get permission to be on my Walk, but perhaps in the future–she will be a blessing whenever and wherever she goes! I am disappointed, but God has other plans for her at this time.

I'm doing report cards this weekend. I only have nine students–7 boys and 2 girls. Four of them are reading at third grade level and have been since Christmas. It keeps me searching for materials as I don't want to put them into the regular books for next year. We are working on chapter books and I keep a few pages ahead to check their comprehension. All my other students are above average too which makes it a joy to teach. I love being able to challenge them. I better enjoy the success now, because next year's group is much lower and quite the challenge with behavior. Oh well! Wait till they get to Mean Old Mrs. McKinney . . .

Keep the e-mails coming, I do appreciate them so much. I am praying for your strength and clear vision of the Kingdom.

Love and prayers,
Judy McK

Bob wrote March 24:

Carol has been in the same state for so long now that sometimes I forget and start to think that she will get better. Then I realize that she still hasn't eaten anything for 26 days. She is a little weaker, but it is such a gradual process that we who are with her every day don't notice it.

She slept all night last night because I was again able to give her the medication at 3:00 A.M. without waking her.

When I realize that she is starving to death, I know that she can't last too much longer, although I still treasure this time we have had together before the Lord takes her home.

I have no regrets as some people have had who haven't been able to tell someone they love that they do love them. The Lord has given me the opportunity to tell her over and over again, that we have had a wonderful life together and that I love her.

For that I am very thankful.

Bob

E-mails received March 24:

It is really good that you are able to share this time. Love to you both.

John & Sue

Bob, I have read your memos, and felt very deeply your pain and anguish these last weeks. Just know that I and many, many more, are praying and praying for Carol and for you, for your strength and courage.

Know that the Lord loves you both very much. SO DO I!!!

Jim Behme

March 25 e-mail from Bob:

Carol didn't sleep well last night. I gave her the normal dose of medicine at 10:00 P.M., which generally keeps her asleep until at least 3:00 A.M.

She woke me up at 1:00 a.m and stayed awake for about an hour. Then she woke up at 4:00 A.M. and stayed awake to about 7:00. I think the medication that we are giving her is wearing off faster. Perhaps she is developing a tolerance to it, I'll have to talk to the hospice nurse tomorrow about it.

Again the frustrating thing when she is awake is to keep moving her so she is in a comfortable position. She has been in bed for 26 days. I'm asking everyone to pray for her comfort and peace. No one knows how long she can keep going without nourishment, so pray that she is comfortable.

Love to all,
Bob

E-mails received March 25:

Dear Bob,

I wonder if it would help Carol to feel more comfortable just to have a slight change in her bedding. I have a foam pad that fits on top of a mattress and under the sheet that is solid on one side and like an egg carton on the other. It should fit fine on a hospital bed. You would be welcome to have it for Carol if you'd like.

Also I wonder if it would fluff and soften her pillows if they were washed. (If they are washable.) Please let me know if I can run by and get them, take them to the laundromat, and return them to you. I know the little things can sometimes help when you are just tired of lying in the same old place. Please let me know if I can help.

Love,
Chris

Dear Bob, our prayers are for Carol but also for YOU! May God grant you courage.

Virginia

We are continuing to lift both of you up in prayer.

God bless,
Dave & Carrie

March 26 e-mail from Bob:

". . . and after you have suffered for a little while, the God of Grace, who has called you to His eternal glory in Christ, will Himself restore, support, strengthen, and establish you. To Him be the power forever and ever, amen" 1 Peter 5:10–11.

49 Days with Hospice

As I read this one of my morning devotions, I couldn't help but think of Carol's suffering.

She said twice today, "I want to go home." She knows she is in our earthly home, so I know she is talking about her heavenly home.

We didn't get much sleep last night. None of the medications we are giving her seem to last as long as they did three weeks ago.

I called Karen Martin, our hospice nurse, and we're waiting now for her to bring some changes in Carol's medications.

What we really need now, however, is a ticket for that trip to her heavenly home.

I've told her many times that even though I love her very much and will miss her, it's all right to go. I love her so much I want her to be with Jesus right now.

The theme of the "Walk to Emmaus" that she lead was, "His sheep I am."

I keep reminding her that Jesus is waiting to pick her up in his arms like a tender lamb and love her.

Pray that she lets go and lets God take her.

In His name,
Bob

Dying with Carol

E-mails received March 26:

> You have been in my prayers and in every group I have been in. Even mopping the floor in the kitchen at Cursillo was done as palanca for the two of you. God bless and keep us aware of your needs.
>
> De Colores
Roger

> Your morning devotion was awesome. I know from experience that if you have given Carol up to the Lord and told her you would be OK, and she is still here, God is doing something that maybe none of us can see. I was reminded by a pastor as I sat at the deathbed of a dear friend, that God will decide when He is going to take her and to look around and see what He is doing. It was amazing, the love that I saw poured out that night. What a blessing that you can look in each other's eyes and continue to affirm your love for each other. I see God in that. I pray for you the strength that you need to complete the task that the Lord has given you in these circumstances and that His peace will surround both of you.
>
> Love in Christ,
Nancy Graf

Tuesday March 27 e-mail from Bob:

> With the help of two nurses, who are good friends, Mary Jane Griffith and Iris DeWilde, I gave a hypodermic shot this morning for her nausea. We changed some of Carol's medications yesterday, upping the strength of some and

trying some directly into her flesh. We have to be careful because Carol is only skin and bones now. She reminds me of some of the Holocaust survivors.

She slept fairly well last night, but it took an hour to get her back to sleep at 1:00 A.M.

I was talking to her about Heaven again during that hour again and I said, "There is nothing to be afraid of" and she answered, "I'm not afraid."

She does appear to me to be somewhat weaker today, but seeing her every day it's hard to judge. It was four weeks ago today that she had her last nourishment intravenously in the hospital.

I told her last night that these last weeks since the end of January when she was in the hospital and now at home are very special to me because of the time we have had together and the many times we have told each other of our love. Sad though it is, I am happy that these last days of our forty-five-year marriage have been a close relationship.

I can really thank the Lord for all things.

Bob

E-mails received March 27:

Dear Bob,

You notes are so tender and to the point. It just brings tears to my eyes.

Dying with Carol

You are a gifted writer.

May that ticket arrive soon.

Love,
Jeanette

Bob:

I must tell you that I pray for you and Carol each day, but I must also tell you that your e-mails to me have ministered to my heart. It is an honor to pray for two people who have shown me so much of what it means to live in faith, even in these very difficult times.

May God sustain you both in every way you need His presence. Some day on the other side we're going to have one whale of a party!

Shalom,
Bruce

Bob

I so much look forward to your daily report about Carol.

May God's loving arms reach down and hold you both.

Dear God, your love encompasses heaven and earth and embraces us everywhere: here, on our journey, and when we come home to You.

Tell Carol–this is the year for the CUBBIES!!!

Mary Merrill

God has given you amazing strength. I'm so glad that you have had this time together.

Blessings.

Sue

Bob's March 28 e-mail:

Yesterday several things happened that tell me that Carol believes her long fight is just about over. When the C.N.A. was giving her a bath, the C.N.A. called me in and said she has something for you. Carol's hand was clenched with something in it. When she opened it to give it to me, it was her wedding rings. She said, "I want you to give this to Robin (our daughter), to give to Acacia. (our grand daughter).

She also has indicated that she knew the end was near. I truly didn't expect her to last the night, but this morning she is still with us, although much weaker.

For those of you who read "The Upper Room" each morning, I wonder how many of you thought of Carol when Paul said in 1 Corinthians 15:42–58 about the body being perishable, but it is raised imperishable and in verse 40, he tells of earthly bodies and heavenly bodies.

I have talked to Carol about the new heavenly body she will have that is free from cancer and all of the discomforts she is going through now.

From the things she has said to me, she is more than ready for this transition. It has reminded me of my mother, who when dying of bone cancer said, "Why is it taking so long?"

Let's all pray that for Carol it doesn't.

Love to all,
Bob

Danny Cox a past pastor of our church has been receiving these e-mails. He asked permission to read some of them in his next Sunday's sermon. He used the e-mails of March 27 & 28. His main point was that only God can provide you with the strength to live through this type of pain and I wholeheartedly agree.

Bob,

You are in our prayers daily. What a loving ordeal you and Carol are experiencing. This Sunday I am preaching about how all our strength, particularly in difficult times, comes from God alone. I would like to read excepts from your writings if you don't mind.

Your faith, and Carol's, show so clearly through your words. I want to share it with others.

Our God Reigns!
Danny

Bob's March 29 e-mail:

Last night between 1:00 A.M. as I waited for Carol to go back to sleep after I gave her the 1:00 A.M. medicine, I started to think about what these e-mail letters mean to me. I guess what I am doing is sharing Carol's dying with you.

I really need the support of all of our friends to face this sad moment in our lives. Carol and I have learned over the years that "The Body of Christ" or the "Church of God" is not just one denomination. Through our Cursillo and Walk to Emmaus experiences, we have met and loved so many strong Christians over the years even inside of prison walls and we know that God doesn't look at where we are, but who we are.

The prayer support that we have received over the last six months is the thing that has carried us through.

When I send this e-mail out I have a file that says, "Carol's Friends." All I have to do is type that into the address of the e-mail and almost 100 people receive this message. We have received over 470 replies from people over the last two months, many of you on a regular basis. It's good to know that during this time you are not alone.

If we did not have this support from our Christian friends, I don't know how I would have been able to handle this.

Thank you for
your love,
Bob

E-mails received March 29:

Bob, when I read your e-mail this A.M. I wanted to share with you again what those e-mails mean to me.

Dying with Carol

Yesterday morning as I was preparing to lead a women's Bible study, I was thinking of the lesson which was on exhortation, or encouragement. I reread again Hebrews 12:18–24 then 13:22.

Shortly after Art's going home, (her husband was killed in an auto accident) when his presence seemed so close to me, I was praying and asked my Lord if those who go on before are really as close as they seem to be. I reached for my Bible and it opened to Hebrews 12:22–24, and Bob, they and we are still as together as we are now. We just cannot touch or see them. We, who belong to Christ are part of the city of the Living God, Ephesians 2:6.

I told the class how those words encourage me in prison ministry, and how now by your e-mails, you are encouraging me in how to die. Thank you Bob and Carol for all you mean to me, for the wonderful love, grace, and courage. The faith you show to all of us.

May the tender love of the Good Shepherd hold you as you as you part for a little while. She will be with Christ and Christ lives in you. You will still be very close.

Love in Christ,
Violet

Dear Bob,

You mentioned how much it has meant to you to share this time with your friends via e-mail. I want you to know it has also meant a great deal to your friends. You have shared your faith valiantly during a terribly challenging time in your life. Although it has broken my heart to know what you and your family have been going through, it has also been a privilege to share this journey in faith with you and to be encouraged by the Lord's faithfulness to you and yours to Him.

Thank you, Bob.

In Jesus,
Chris

More March 29 e-mails:

Dear Bob and Carol,

I have so much appreciated the e-mails and being considered one of your friends. You both have meant more to me than you will ever realize. You both supported me so much during a very dark valley in my life. That's what friends are for and I am so glad to be able to support you in prayer during this time. I think of you both often every day and send up prayers that you will both have the peace of Jesus that surpasses all understanding.

Carol, I am so glad that I have a room in your big yellow mansion. We'll sing God's praises together once again.

Love,
Cindy

Dying with Carol

I feel really badly that I have been receiving all your e-mails thru friends but have failed to respond to you in your time of need, Bob. Please forgive me.

There is no way I can feel your pain and loss as you go thru this, but I want you to know that how you are dealing/handling this is a great inspiration to me. Ever since you called to tell me you could not be on my team, we have had a very special relationship and you have been a special friend to me. And you always will be. May our Lord be with you throughout this time, and comfort you and strengthen you and bless you for the time(s) you and Carol had together.

God bless you, my very special friend.

> OMG (that's "Old Man Gray,"
> otherwise Gary Gray)

Bob,

We read your message every day and Carol and your family are continually in our prayers. We don't know why God is dragging this on so long for her but there must be a reason. As you said in one of your earlier messages 'Let go and let God'. We hope her suffering ends soon. We will continue to pray.

> God bless
> John and Darlene Wood

Dear Bob,

Your e-mail really touched my heart as I feel much the same way about the body of Christ and the people we've met and loved through Emmaus–that includes the two of you. It doesn't make any difference what denomination we are or you are, we love because hopefully, the love of our Lord flows through each of us. If sharing has been a help to you, we praise God and give Him the glory, in the sharing we have also been blessed.

May the peace of God rest on both of you.

Nancy and Karl Graf

Bob's March 30 e-mail:

The only request Carol has made of us, other than minor adjustments in her bed position, is to be hugged.

Many of you know Carol as the Dr. of Huggology, a skit we used to put on during Walk to Emmaus weekends. Especially now during this time we all need a hug, and especially Carol.

Would you do me a favor today? Find someone and give them a hug and tell them it's for Carol Lillie. You may have to explain the circumstances, but that's all right too.

I'm sure Carol would be pleased to know she again got her Christian friends to hug one another. If anyone would like a copy of that skit let me know and I'll e-mail it to you.

A hug to all,
Bob

Dying with Carol

E-mails received March 30:

> Yes, we would like a copy of your and Carol's skit. Isn't that tender that she is still alert enough and sensitive enough to want and need a hug. Mr. Kassing will be the recipient of the hug!
>
> Love,
The Kassings
>
> Hugs are a'comin! And you know, she will soon be getting hugs from the one whose arms we have all longed to feel. Blessings to you both.
>
> Sue

Sent Friday, March 30, 2001, 10:30 AM:

> Bob when you have a chance mail me a copy of the hug skit. There is a man in our a cappella choir at church–a recovering alcoholic who is always ready to hug and be hugged. I'll give him a Carol Hug tonight.
>
> Virginia

> Dearest Bob,
>
> I would love a copy of that skit. Last night as I said my prayers, I asked why it is taking Carol so long to get to heaven. I suddenly felt surrounded by people and then I realized that they we all friends of Carol's. They were all witnessing the ultimate "love of God." Carol and your love, faith and trust is an amazing lesson to everyone that knows you or knows of you. None of us will ever

forget what you have gone through and how your grace has shone through adversity every single day.

We have only had the privilege of knowing you two for a couple of years, but the lesson we've learned from you will last us the rest of our lives.

Please give Carol a hug from us (me, Don and Bethany). This has been a wonderful example of true Christian faith for our 10 year old, too.

Our love and prayers continue for you and your family.

> Bless you.
> The Shuford family,
> Cindy, Don, and Bethany

I will hug my kids and friends today in honor of my friend Carol Lillie. Please let her know I am hugging her too, in my heart. I would love to have the copy of that skit. Bless you for your love and endurance during what must be a very trying time. I pray for all of you that it is over soon and Carol goes to that Heavenly Home.

> Love,
> JoEtta

Bob's March 31 e-mail:

A few days ago I concluded the e-mail with "Thank the Lord." After I wrote it, I started to think about all of the things I should thank God for, even though our family is going through this time of trial.

Dying with Carol

First, I thank the Lord that Carol is not in a lot of pain. She is uncomfortable from lying so long in a bed, but she isn't in the pain I saw my mother go through dying of bone cancer.

Second, I thank the Lord for my family, my two wonderful kids who love their mother and love me.

I also thank the Lord for Carol's brother and his wife who are staying with me during this time.

Next, I thank the Lord for all of our Christian friends who are praying for us and going through this time with us.

Then, I thank the Lord that he has given Carol and I 45 years together with the joys and sorrows we have experienced together.

Finally, and most of all, I thank the Lord for the faith he has given us, so that we both know that there is a heavenly home and a new body waiting for us. We really believe that the Lord has directed our lives for these 45 years and led us to the great joy of His agape love.

Carol is each day showing the signs that the end is near. When she is awake she stares at the ceiling most of the time with her eyes apparently fixed on nothing.
She still knows everyone and there appears to be a greater peace settling over her than we have seen in the last few weeks. I hope when my time on earth comes to an end, I experience the peace that I see in Carol now.

Love to all,
Bob

49 Days with Hospice

E-mails received March 31:

Dear Bob,

Gary and I just got home today. We were in Florida for two weeks. I had asked Marilyn to call and let us know how Carol was doing. I just read your messages and I am amazed that her body can take what is happening to her.

You and Carol and the rest of your family have been in our constant prayers.

I know this has got to be very difficult for you to see someone you love so much go through what Carol is going through. I intend to give out lots of hugs tomorrow at church for Carol. She gave great hugs and I enjoyed her Dr. Hug skit. I remember when she gave it at the prison and the girls enjoyed it so much. We will give the ladies at Dwight hugs this weekend in Carol's name. We finally got our clearance to go in this coming weekend. As you share with us each day what is going on with Carol, just know how much it means to Gary and I that you would share such a personal part of your life with those who love the two of you so much.

I lost my Mom a year ago on April 1 and that was so hard, but I'm thankful she didn't have to suffer a long time. She also had ovarian cancer. May the peace of Christ be with both of you. God's blessings to you.

Love in Christ.

Gary & Linnie

Dying with Carol

April 1 e-mail from Bob:

> Three times in the last 24 hours, I was sure that Carol was going to leave us. One time was when she was hugging our son, Bob, who drove in from Louisville, KY to be with us for a few hours. She told him twice she was going to die, and he told her it was all right. The last time was at 5:00 A.M. this morning when I was giving her some medicine. She seemed to come right up to the doors of death and then for some reason stepped back. It can't be too long before she takes that final step. The physical signs are mostly all there, but for some reason God is letting her tarry.
>
> I went to church again this morning while Bob and his wife, Jennifer and Carol's brother and his wife, Marty, stayed home with her.
>
> We had communion this morning and as always partaking in the Body and Blood of our Lord was what I really needed. Especially at this time.
>
> In Jeremiah it says, "I know the plans I have for you," says the Lord. There are times I wish I knew what those plans are. Our pastor this morning reminded me that one of the fruits of the Spirit is patience. I must dig down deep into that fruit during this time. As a lay leader in the Walk to Emmaus, I had to give a talk called "Perseverance." I'll have to re-read that talk.
>
> Love to all,
> Bob

49 Days with Hospice

E-mails received April 1:

Dear Bob,

This morning's sermon was a very difficult one for me. After knowing you and Carol so well and after all the two of you have done for me, I couldn't help thinking–I hope in some small way I can be a witness of Jesus' love to others as you and Carol have been to me and to so many, many people.

Frank recorded Danny's sermon for you. The sound is good, but the picture is real fuzzy. I am trying to locate a better copy from the TV crew.

I am sure you will all be very pleased about how Danny used your experiences to illustrate how powerless we are without God–but how he can empower us to do so much.

I will get a tape to you sometime this week.

In Jesus' love,
Cindy

We taped Danny's message for you–would you like us to mail you the tape or bring it over sometime? It was a good message–he read a few of your recent e-mails and talked about having strength in the Lord. May you continue to be strong, now and even after Carol goes home to be with our Lord. She is the lucky one–she awaits her eternal reward we all have to d eal with being without her and still being here on earth to finish whatever work God still has for us to do! Give her a hug from Tom and me.

Dying with Carol

Love ya both.

Linda

April 2 e-mail from Bob:

It's unbelievable that Carol is still holding on. Tomorrow it will be 5 weeks since she has had any nourishment. She is still aware what is going on and responds to people. Another worry has popped up, because her stomach is swelling the way it did when we first detected the ovarian cancer. My prayer is that it doesn't attack something that will cause her to be in pain.

I've received so many e-mails telling of people giving someone a hug for Carol. I know that even in dying, Carol still has a ministry going on to spread God's agape love across the world.

One way I have known that we have been empowered by the Holy Spirit is by our agape love for so many people over the years. One thing I know is, you can't be jealous when the love your wife is showing to others is God's agape love. Paul said in the thirteenth chapter of First Corinthians that the greatest of the gifts of the spirit is agape love. I know Carol has that gift.

Her ministry of hugs even worked behind prison walls. I want you all to pray for our many friends who are going into Dwight Correctional Center next weekend. Normally Carol and I would be on that team.

God loves you
and

49 Days with Hospice

We love you,
Bob

E-mails received April 2:

Bob,

James and I are leaving for Florida tomorrow and won't be back until the 25th. My mother's health is fragile and she needs some help. She was in the hospital for a week with acute bronchitis and now is in a rehab/nursing home facility. Well enough to leave the hospital but not well enough to come home.

I have enjoyed reading your e-mails. They are filled with love for Carol and a heart that can rejoice in this time. We pray for you, your family, and especially for Carol daily. You are always close to our thoughts. I most likely won't be able to be at Carol's funeral, but I want you to know that I will be there in the spirit, praying for you and the family. Please, please give Carol our love and we hugged one another the other day for Carol. And please receive the hug and love we are sending you. I am so glad that the Lord brought our paths together. Carol's suffering has made me think about a lot of things and to think that she is so close to the throne of God and to being healed is, well, mind boggling. Praise the Lord!

Love,
Paula and family

Dying with Carol

Dear Bob,

I am glad to hear that Carol's hug ministry is carrying on. I, too, found people to hug at the track meet Friday afternoon. They turned out to be people who love you and Carol as I do.

Love Ya!
Marj

Another April 2 e-mail:

I'm getting ready to go to our Group Reunion meeting–Pat Kelly, Chuck and I meet on Monday evenings at McDonald's in Creve Couer. Our prayers will be for you and Carol.

I just want you to know (again) how much I appreciate your e-mails. Through each bit of information from you, I relive my father-in-law's last days. He died just a couple of weeks ago. It helps me to see your words, to know of your commitment to Jesus Christ and to know that Carol is in His hands–just as I knew my father-in-law was. What do people do who don't know Jesus?

We love both you and Carol–we know He loves both of you.

Jim Behme

Give my love to Carol. Please tell her we are with her every bit of her difficult journey with hugs and prayers.

We shall follow her path forever. She is forever in our daily thoughts. And so are you, Bob, and thanks for all your daily news and sharing with us. I had a long phone call and visit with Doris last week. I had my 65th birthday and she called. Her nickel this time. She is one very busy lady and involved with a lot of national women's group. She even had a visit to Israel last year that proved to be very educational as far as what is REALLY HAPPENING behind the scenes.

Yes, we sure gave a lot of hugs around this area and with each other. Don't we wish we could all help Carol! I hope she is not in pain and not swelling any more.

We love you, we pray for you!

Jacquinot and Bob

April 3 e-mail from Bob:

Tuesday April 3rd

Carol woke up at 4:00 A.M. this morning and really had a bad time. She was is so much discomfort from her stomach swelling with the ovarian cancer fluid. I was finally able to move her into a position that was more comfortable and she was able to get some sleep.
I spoke with the hospice nurse this afternoon and we will probably be shortening the time periods between her medication.

Dying with Carol

Thirty-five days without any nourishment is a long time. I wonder how thin Jesus got in his 40 days in the wilderness.

I saw an ad on television on television about a show called "The Fighting Fitzgerald's." The father was being asked how he mourned his wife's death. He said something I have thought of many times. "She wasn't supposed to die before me. I was supposed to go first."
All my life with insurance and many other things, I assumed that I would go before Carol, not the other way around.

I just pray now that God will take her out of this state that she is in and take her home.

Please join me in
that prayer,
Bob

April 3 e-mails received:

Bob,

That [hug] skit makes me think of the two of you so much!

I would very much like the words to it and if you would allow us to, my husband Stanley and I, would like to borrow that wonderful ministry from you for the time being. Talk it over with Carol and ask her if that would be all right with her. We would include Carol and you in the skit somehow to let everyone know that these are hugs from you too.

I pray for Carol, you and your family daily.

In Christ,
Eva Marie White

Bob,

We are praying constantly. I so hope she is home with her Lord real soon.

I wake up so many times at night thinking she must be in trouble and pray for you guys. All our love.

P.S. Our little Meredith is in the hospital with an asthma attack since yesterday morning. Hope she gets home soon.

Mike & Ilona

The following beautiful prayer came April 3 from a good friend Carolyn Schoof:

Faithful Father in Heaven,

I give you praise this night Lord, for you are Holy, Just and Loving. You, oh Lord, have given us the most splendid gift a father could ever give to his children. You have given us the power to receive eternal life by simply believing in Jesus as our Savior and repenting of our many sins. Thank you for your love and care for us. Thank you for planning a way for us to be able to be with you when our days on this earth are over. We look forward to being with you in the beautiful home that Jesus said he was going to prepare for all of us.

Father, in the name of your son Jesus, I come to intercede for my sister in Christ, Carol. I thank you for the many years of friendship that we have shared. I thank you for the beautiful example of a mother that she has been for my own son through the years. I thank you for the many times that she has lifted my name before you in prayer. I thank you for the beautiful voice that she shared with the choir and our church for so many years. She never grew tired of lifting your name in praise. I thank you for the beautiful example she has shown and lived in being a devoted wife to Bob.

Thank you for the wonderful years that they have shared together. I thank you for the splendid gift of painting that Carol freely shared with all she has known. Thank you for the gift of courage that you have given to her to be able to witness for you before so many people. Thank you also for the love she gave so freely to the women and men she has met in the prisons as she testified for you.

What a blessing to have had her for a secret prayer pal. She certainly let you know that you were loved. Lord, right now she needs your presence with her. She is waiting for you to come and receive her unto yourself. I ask that Satan be bound and cast from her and Bob's home. That any fears she may have would be stilled and would disappear.

Again I know that if it be your will, you could and would still heal her completely by the power of Jesus' name. But I would ask for your will to be done right now and not mine. It is hard to let go of the ones we love so much. Quiet our own hearts from fear and loneliness. Thank you for letting us know that you are near. I can't help but think maybe you are waiting for Easter, so we may rejoice not only for the resurrection of our Savior but also for the resurrection of our dear Carol.

You are God and you have promised to be with us all the time. Please come be with us now. In the name of our Beloved Savior, Jesus. Amen.

You've got the prayers, and the Bible studies of this church are also praying for you.
Blessings.

Sue

Bob's April 4 e-mail:

Our hospice nurse, Karen Martin, asked me yesterday if Carol was hanging on for some special reason. Five weeks without nourishment is a very long time and she wondered what was keeping Carol going.

I've asked Carol several times if she is ready and she has always said "Yes."

The only thing we can ascertain is her body, heart, and lungs are still strong enough to maintain life.

She again is showing some signs of failing and just now when the C.N.A. asked her how she was, she said, "Rotten."

Dying with Carol

We shortened the period between her medications and we are increasing some of it on the advice of her ovarian cancer doctor. I think most of her discomfort is because the ovarian cancer is causing her stomach cavity to fill the way it did when it was first detected.

Please Lord, take her before the pain gets too great.

In Jesus name,
Bob

The following e-mails came in April 4:

Prayers continue that God would take Carol home ASAP (His time). We just never know how life is going to turn out. You are doing a good job, Bob.

You are loved,
The Kassings

Dear Bob,

I know it must be terribly hard to see and understand what is going on with Carol. I am at a loss of what to say other than I love you both very much and I know that the Lord has good things in store for you.

Love,
Cindy

Just sending you all an electronic hug.

Bob, as I read about your concern about Carol's lack of nourishment as we know it . . . I'm sure it is bothering you far more than her. Years ago, I cared for a gentleman who was in the last stages of abdominal cancer. At the time, the thinking was to continue to try to give the body nourishment in the form of human food for "strength." The result was horrendous. I will spare you the details.

You are giving Carol the real nourishment she needs now. Love and more love. And being the channel to share all the love being sent to her from the rest of us.

As I have prayed and reflected on the great gift of our Savior, it occurred to me that Carol may be waiting for Easter.

Love,
Margo

Bob,

Just a short note to let all of you know that you are still in our prayers. It is not an easy time and it can be really frustrating to watch someone you love linger on and on. If there is anything I can do, please feel free to ask.

In His Love,
Pat Monroe

April 5 e-mail from Bob:

Carol is getting weaker every day. Her increased medication keeps her sleeping most of the time and in many ways that is a blessing.

Dying with Carol

Our pastor has to be out of town the afternoon of the 8th until late on the 11th. He has another minister to fill in for him, but that man doesn't know Carol. I'd really hate to have someone do the service who doesn't know her.

Maybe I shouldn't be thinking about things like this, but our life has been so centered around our church, that I want Carol's final goodbye to be perfect.

I've got our pastor's permission to call another United Methodist pastor if I need to because he understands my point and agrees with it.

We'll have to delay any plans until our daughter, Robin, can get back here from Phoenix.

I hope you all can understand my acceptance of Carol's eventual death. We have had 45 good years together and I don't want to have her last days with us be in a lot of pain. Our faith assures us that she will have a new body, free from cancer and pain.

Maybe these last few weeks have been to bring me to this acceptance.

I thank you all for sharing them with me.

Love to all,
Bob

The following e-mails were received April 5:

Dearest Bob:

Our hearts are with you. My e-mail hasn't worked for several months, but came home tonight determined. This is what I found from a Team Member of Walk #14. This is what you and Carol helped Bob and I find in the Emmaus Movement.

God Bless,
Alice and Bob Williamson

Bob,

I totally understand your concern about someone that doesn't know Carol doing the service. I hope it makes you smile to know that about 10 years ago, I got very concerned about what music would be played at my funeral. I could picture Jim saying, "It doesn't matter–anything will do." I am figuring that I would be "someplace" saying, "It does too matter!!!" So I wrote my top choices in the back of a music book. Jen knows just where to find it. If Jim even thinks about saying "It doesn't matter . . ." Jen will whip out the book.

You are in my prayers.

Love Ya!
Marj

Dying with Carol

Dear Bob,

Your realness and honesty is so refreshing. Can certainly understand how you'd want to have your pastor give Carol's funeral service. Prayers to you all, to keep on keeping on.

With love,
The Kassings

Dear Bob,

I have read your e-mails every day and I have been keeping you in my prayers. I do believe that God knows the right timing for everyone, not only the one who is dying. I have felt so close to what you are going through because of my own experience. No two circumstances are ever the same but I am sure we have shared a lot of the same feelings in dealing with our loved ones. Losing Tammy and Dad were both very hard but completely different. Isn't it wonderful to know that they and Carol knew their heavenly Father so well. That is such a comfort. I will continue to keep you all in my daily prayers as the days become more difficult. I have found, as I'm sure you will with time, that by letting God use me to help others in similar circumstances, it's the best way I've been able to find healing for myself.

Please don't hesitate to ask if Roger or I can do anything to help you now or later.

In His Precious Love
Elaine

April 6 e-mail from Bob:

Last night around 9:00 P.M., we really thought Carol was going to leave us. We gathered around her, her brother, her sister-in law, her good friend Jane, and me. Her breathing was very irregular and her pulse was rapid and weak. In many ways, we all said good-bye to her. About 11:00 P.M. I told the others that they had better get some sleep because I would need them the next day. I watched her on and off through the night and at daylight she was still with us. When I talked to our hospice nurse, Karen Martin, at 8:00 A.M., I asked her to bring enough medication for the weekend, just to be safe.

This morning as I was giving her a kiss; she put her hand behind my head and held it close to her for over a minute. Then she smiled.

I don't know what God's timing is, but as I have said before, I thank Him for these precious moments of the last 12 weeks.

In 45 years of marriage, unfortunately, you take your love for your spouse for granted. These days together have renewed that very tender love I may have forgotten.

Carol, I don't believe, has any concept of what day it is or how long this has been going on. Sunday will be 40 days since she has had any nourishment. The same fast Our Lord did before he started his ministry.

Love to all,
Bob

Dying with Carol

April 6 e-mails received:

Bob:

What a beautiful story your shared today, of tenderness and shared life. Today is my wife's 50th birthday, and I am going to make sure she knows when her head hits the pillow tonight that she is a gift from God to me.

May his love sustain you in these days. Tell Carol I love her. Then remember that I love you, too.

Bruce

Dear Bob,

We have been out at a prayer ministry school and couldn't contact you. We wanted you to know that we continue to hold you in our prayers. We were at our son's when you sent the message about the hugs. That was in New Jersey, but got my e-mail on his computer. Just as God would plan, isn't it that I told Scott and his wife about Carol and then gave Scott and Susan and Karl my hugs for her. I'm a hugger too so that wasn't too difficult.

Will continue to keep you and your family in my prayers. Only God knows why she is still with us, but He has a purpose. My computer is broken so am using Karl's laptop and am not very good at it. Excuse the errors.

We love you in the Lord and we send a hug to you.

Love,
Nancy Graf

49 Days with Hospice

Bob's April 7 e-mail:

Carol is asleep about 98% of the time today. We're still able to give her the medication, but have to be careful that she doesn't choke on it. When she is awake, she still knows what is going on and can respond with a single word. At least she isn't aware of the discomfort that we know about. She can't go on much longer, although the nurse said yesterday, when she listened to her heart and lungs, that if she didn't know how long she had been without nourishment. She would think another week or so.

The nurse also said, if we had kept her on the tube feeding, she probably would be gone by now. Her reasoning is that the cancer has been starved by the lack of nourishment and for that reason is slower growing.
When I'm with her in the middle of the night, I watch her chest to see if it is still occasionally going up and down. Sometimes you can hear her breathing, but not always.

She has so many times come to the edge of passing on and then comes back; it is hard to predict. I guess this is what they call living on the edge.

We're truly in God's hands.

Love to all,
Bob

Dying with Carol

April 7 e-mails received:

Bob,

As I prayed on the way home–I knew that all the people in Dwight Correctional Center were praying, too. There are so many who love and adore Carol. I wouldn't have known Carol, I'm afraid. I never had seen her with gray hair.

I hope she heard the words I whispered to her, though. She has been such an inspiration to so many. I just hope all of us who crossed her path can carry on her "HUG-OLOGY" ministry among the many others she inspired. I consider it such a privilege to have been on 4 teams with her–3 of them with you, too at Dwight.

The first time I was with her, I was a new Table Leader on Walk 80 with another lady. Carol was giving the priority talk. She really took me under her wing as I ended up with a very difficult person at my table. She supported me and taught me and I knew from then on that my Emmaus family was something very special. Last fall, on Mary Jane's team, we were cut short of her tremendous talent.

Thank you again, for continuing to let us hear how each day progresses. It means so much to have shared parts of her life and now the days of her death.

Love and Prayers,
Judy McK

49 Days with Hospice

Bob's April 8 e-mail:

It's been 40 days since Carol has had any nourishment. Last night as I was sitting next to her watching her breathing. I thought about Jesus fasting for 40 days before he started his ministry. How weak and thin he must have been. That's probably why the devil thought he could tempt him.

Carol is getting weaker every day. I'm glad so far she hasn't had any real pain.

Another thing I want to share with you is that the Lord works in mysterious ways, even with our Internal Revenue Service. Carol's brother, Clete and his wife have been here over a month and they came on short notice. Clete started to get worried about filing his income tax next week. He hadn't done it yet. His son Steve called a few days ago and told him because of the devastating fires in New Mexico last year, the Federal Government has given those counties exemptions from filing until January of 2002.

Clete said they were 80 miles away from the fires, but for some reason his county was included. That has to be a miracle from God. Who else could affect the IRS?
I really want you to pray for him and his wife Marty. They have really hung in there with me. I don't know what I would have done without them.

God does provide!
Bob

Dying with Carol

April 8 e-mails received:

Dearest Bob

As this Holy Week unfolds, know that you are loved and uplifted in prayer by many. Carol has always been one of God's special servants and as we know all to well, the road is never smooth, but He is with us. Why so long? We may never know this side of heaven–I pray for you a sense of peace. Peace that comes only from God.

The decisions that were made for Carol were the best that you could make at the time (feeding tube or not). Modern medicine is great, but God is in control, as you well know.

Easter Week is a special time for Dick and myself. We both lost our mothers during this time. I lost mine on Good Friday in 1987 and Dick lost his mother four years ago with the funeral on Friday before Palm Sunday.

Knowing that we will see our loved ones again and Easter season reinforcing that is still a great blessing. Who knows, maybe that's why Carol has been allowed to stay so that she may come home during the greatest week of the year.

We have an awesome God–whose timing is perfect. God bless you and yours during this wonderful season.

With all our love,
Dick and Christa

Again, thanks for sharing various miracles. Interesting hearing how things would have been different with the tube feeding? Yes, you all are living on the edge, but trusting in God in the process. What a labor of love your relatives have provided.

Prayers continue.

The Kassings

Dear Bob,

I don't know that your remember me but I was married 10 years ago to Jim _____. Angela _____ is our daughter.

Jim and I have been in touch with each other for about one year. He lives in Eureka and I now live in AZ.
I have been reading your e-mails and they have really made me realize that he and I need to work on our relationship together. I recently came back and we went to see a Christian counselor in Peoria. I am going to step out on faith and come back to go to counseling with Jim.

I love it here and love my friends and my job. I don't like Eureka as it has never been someplace I have wanted to live. But listening to you talk about your love for your wife and your love of Christ, I feel that I need to come back and be committed to counseling.

We still love one another. I love him but I want him to want to come to AZ. Jim says I should love him no matter where he is. He should be first in my life, not AZ.

I thank you for your help in the past weeks and know that I am praying for you.

Dying with Carol

Bob's Monday, April 9 e-mail:

Thank God Carol's not in any pain. She looks so pitiful lying there on her hospital bed. She is still very much aware of what is going on around her.

Karen, our hospice nurse, keeps thinking she will fall into a coma, but that hasn't happened yet. She is so beautiful. Maybe God is trying to show me how unappreciative I have been of my wife of 45 years. Maybe he wants me to miss her more when she is gone.

Like most married couples, we had our differences. During these weeks at home and in the hospital, we have lived in perfect agreement with one another. Isn't it too bad that it had to be in dying that this takes place. We all know men and women have different ways at looking at life. Perhaps with Carol and I, it is looking at death that brings us into final agreement.

Her heart goes on. Now I really know what a strong women I married. Our children may have to worry about the legacy of cancer they are inheriting, but they also should know that they are inheriting a strong heart and a will to live from their mother.

We are so rich in Christian friends. We can't leave them to our children in our wills, but we can leave them an example that they are witnessing now as their mother dies.

We are the richest couple on the face of the earth.

Love,
Bob

April 9 e-mails received:

Good Morning!

Hope you had a good night. Bob, you looked tired and I pray you got a good night of rest. We are sorry we delayed your supper. We did not realize it was that late. It is so hard to leave when you know it could be the last time Carol is there. It would be the best for all of you though if it can be soon, because it will soon take a toll on all of you. I admire you all how well you are handling all of the situations you are put in. Fantastic job.

That singer was really great and such a sweet person. (Carolyn Schoof came and sang "Wind Beneath My Wings" for Carol from me.)

Well I must get the laundry going. God bless you all and God is really working in shaping all of us for the last day and his coming.

Love to all,
M & I

Bob:

Thank you for sharing that e-mail. It is very special. Even in these very hurtful days, God is using your circumstances to reach out to others.

To paraphrase what Joseph told his brothers, "What Satan meant for evil, God used for good."

Amen.

Dying with Carol

I pray for you and Carol and your family every day. If I can do anything at all to help you, please let me know.

Shalom,
Bruce

Bob, thank you for this. It shows that God is at work in your difficult situation to bring uncounted blessings to others.

You, Carol and all remain close in our prayers.
Our God reigns.

Danny

Tuesday April 10 e-mail from Bob:

It's been 6 weeks since Carol has had any nourishment and still she is with us and is aware what is happening to her.

Hospice is just giving us a day's supply of her medication at a time because they are also surprised that she is hanging on so long. I can understand that because the cost of the medication is well over $100.00 a day. They can't take back any that is left over. I wonder if God will ever reveal to us what his purpose is in having Carol survive for this long a period.

I have seen some reasons by some of the e-mails I am getting in response. One is of a broken marriage, that God willing, might be restored.

I guess, in many ways, Carol's dying process is teaching us all a little something about facing our own deaths some day.

She is less and less responsive, although, as I have said before, she still knows us and responds in some way to us.

I can't say enough for our sister-in law, Marty Blunier. She is really an angel in human form, for both of us. The support of our church and all of our Christian friends has been a true blessing.

God loves you all and so do I.

                                                                Bob

E-mails received April 10:

Dear Bob,

Every day I expect to hear the sad news that Carol has gone to be with her angels, but somehow her heart and body is not ready to give up being with you and her loved ones. I pray that she and all of you are not suffering.

Emotionally you all must be on a train heading out into a vast no man's land, wondering what it all means. Thank goodness you have been able to have these special moments and hours together. It is so difficult
to absorb what all of you are going through. I know you are going to be one lonely man when Carol leaves this life, especially since every moment of each day you have been at her side. You will need to make some plans to be

with some loved ones so that the emptiness in the house doesn't take you into the pits of depression. You know that we are with you in heart, mind, and prayers every day.

Thank goodness you have so many right there in Eureka that can help you with food and anything else that is needed during this time. Thank goodness for our little town. Aren't you glad that you didn't make that move to Florida several years ago when you were thinking of building on that land that you purchased? Guess there is a purpose for everything. Hard to see it sometimes! I hope that you are ok, and have the strength to see the final closure. I am so glad that you have some wonderful friends and that Cletus and Marty can be there during all this time. Brothers Bob and Gene also send their love to you, and so does my Bob!

He tells me of his love every day–many times. We are blessed. My love and prayers to Carol!

Love,
Jacquinot

Dear Bob,

Watch and see if you can see things that the Lord is doing. Some of it, He is doing through you. You've shown courage and strength and wisdom and love in the most trying circumstances. Only God can do that through you. I know in all cases that God will take the person when HE is ready and until then He is working through both of you to glorify Himself and bring glory and honor to His kingdom. He is using you both in a most unusual way and I'm sure over the years to come, you will find out some of the things He is doing. Then some of the things you probably won't learn until you get to heaven. May He bless you with all the GOOD things He has for you and may His strength keep you going from now until the day of His coming.

Love in Jesus,
Nancy Graf

Wednesday, April 11 e-mail from Bob:

The nurse said this morning that Carol's pulse was very weak and her blood pressure was 91 over 63. Her skin is also showing some signs that the end is near.

Carol, seems rather complacent waiting for the end. She speaks to us rather quietly and still can answer questions mainly about water. I've seen people pass away before, but never in slow motion as Carol seems to be doing. Even Karen, our hospice nurse has said this is very rare.

As I have said before, I'm so thankful that she is not in any apparent pain. Whenever we ask her she says, "No." We can still tell each other we love one another, and I guess that is the most important thing.

In Jesus' time the Greeks had 5 or 6 words for love. Carol and I have experienced several of them. But at this stage of our lives, I think, we share agape love or the type of love that expects nothing in return. It is that kind of love that would want a loved one to leave this life and go live with God.

Maybe that is why it has taken so long. My greatest wish for Carol now is to be with God in heaven.

Please pray this with me,
Bob

E-mails received April 11:

Dear Bob,

Thanks for sending the e-mails from Tami. Please be assured that I pray for you and Carol and the whole family many times a day. Your love for the Lord and for Carol has indeed touched my life as it has many others.

Love,
Cindy

Thursday April 12 e-mail from Bob:

Carol's body seems to now be rejecting even the limited amount of water we have been giving her. Last night at 7:00 P.M. and then this morning at 5:00 A.M., she vomited up all of the fluids that she had in her stomach. It appears that the cancer has again produced another bowel blockage. She is also complaining about some pain in her stomach. We are going to try to control this with suppositories rather than oral medicines. Because of her colostomy, we can do it without disturbing her or waking her up.

This is Carol's brother and his wife's 42nd wedding anniversary. I am so grateful that they can be here to help take care of her.

Much to the surprise of the hospice people, Carol still is aware of everything and recognizes us and speaks to us on a limited basis.

We are going to try to appease her thirst with just a small sponge of water rather than allowing her to sip from a straw. This is because she drinks too fast and that causes the nausea. With her water restricted and no nourishment, how long can she hang on? We pray that we are making the right decisions for her comfort during her final hours.

Keep praying
Bob

April 12 e-mails received:

Dear Bob,

Yes, you are making the right decisions. You are praying and doing the best you know how. You have continued to do the best you know how—how can ANYONE do more than that. You will never have to regret not caring for Carol in the best way you knew how. God has extended much grace to you, to Cletus and to Marty to enable you to do just that.

You are all in my prayers.

Jesus loves you and so do I.

Cindy

Dying with Carol

Bob:

Thanks for the updates. Our hearts & prayers go out to you, Carol & family. We know it has to be so tough on all of you, but as He always does, the Lord gives you the strength to handle it.

It's incredible how she has hung on so long. Obviously, she and the Lord have their own plans. Donna, my sister, fooled the nurses also by lasting longer than she should have. She was fighting her way to a Sunday & she made it. Maybe Carol wants to make it to the Easter weekend. What a glorious time to go home to the Lord that would be.

If there is anything at all we can do for you, please let us know. In the meantime, our prayers continue for all of you.

The Lord's will be done.

God bless you all, Bob. Some eternal generational blessings are occurring now for you and everyone else involved in this. Even amongst the suffering you and Carol are enduring.

Always thinking of you,
Sherry

Hi Bob,

I just wanted to let you know how much your e-mails encourage me. It is neat for "newlyweds" like Dave and I to see how much you still love Carol after 45 years. I find that very encouraging and uplifting.

> Love in Christ,
> Carrie

Bob,

You and all your loved ones are very much on our minds as we go through this Holy Week.

Thank you, thank you for sharing your painful struggle to Calgary.

> Love Ya!
> Marj

Friday, April 13 e-mail from Bob:

(Good Friday)

I held off writing this today because I thought I'd have a different message. Carol spent a good part of last night vomiting and this morning by 5:00 A.M. we really thought it was over. Carol also thought it also. One thing she said is, "Is why is it taking so long?" The same thing my mother said twenty years ago before she passed away from bone cancer.

Carol and I said the Lord's Prayer together and her breathing was very shallow and by the time the hospice nurse got here at 7:30. She could not find her pulse. We gave her a shot for her nausea and some sleeping medicine and she calmed down and now at almost 5:00 P.M. she is still with us.

All our hospice nurse, Karen, can say is, "She is one tough lady."

All of us here, her brother, Clete, and his wife, Marty, and I are quite tired. I can only pray that she will pass away quietly in her sleep. I really thought Good Friday might be the day and maybe it still will be. God's grace is the only thing that can keep us going through this long process. Even Carol is tired of it and wants to go. She keeps telling me she's not afraid and I know that is true.

Pray for her peace.

Bob

E-mails received April 13:

We continue to pray for all of you. It would be indeed symbolic if Carol were to go home during this Holy weekend.

Virginia

Easter Saturday e-mail from Bob:

I know God has a reason for stretching Carol's death out so long. So far she hasn't had any real pain, but there are some sores she has on her backside that look to be possibly very painful.

Last night at 2:30 A.M. she said "I want to go home" again. We both prayed that the Lord would take her. Her blood pressure this morning was 91 over 71 and her heartbeat was 148. She did get a little sick when the C.N.A. was bathing her this morning, but other than that the shots and suppositories have been controlling her nausea.

Her good friend, Jane Griffith, a nurse, came and gave her the shot this morning. She is not taking any morphine any more because the water she needs with it makes her vomit. I hope nothing I am doing is causing our Lord to keep Carol here.

We have been through a lot of things together during our forty-five year marriage. But now I find myself praying that it will end.

"Lord, please give Carol the peace she is asking for. But not our will, but your will be done. "

Bob

April 14 e-mail received:

Dear Bob and Carol

Our prayers are with you, today, and all of the days since you have been struggling through this daily ordeal. Even though I haven't been able to get on the computer every day, you are in my thoughts all the time. I can't imagine how this has been for all of you every hour of the day and every minute. It must be hard for Cletus to realize he is losing his second sister from cancer. It will be Easter tomorrow, maybe this will be the day that Carol will be with our Lord and all her little angels. I surely hope so because I don't understand how she could possibly go through any more. Sure hard to understand.

Dying with Carol

Today was a beautiful day here so I worked out in my garden. I pulled up some carrots, beets, parsnips, and onions that I had grown last summer. Since we don't get super cold freezes here during the winter, we can leave the root crops in the soil and use as needed. Tonight we had some fresh carrots and parsnips to go with some sauerkraut, meat, and potatoes.

Sure tasted good. Since we are having a drought this summer (unless something drastically changes with our rain) I am wondering how much of a garden to put in. We may have only enough to drink and bathe. Time will tell.

When I think about gardens, I think about Carol and how excited she was to plant her roses, bulbs, and others. She was a hard worker and quite an artist.

My love to all of you, my prayers and love to Carol. May Carol not suffer any longer and soon be with her angels!

Jacquinot and Bob, too!!!!

Easter Sunday e-mail from Bob:

We're all pretty tired today. We were up with Carol from 1:30 A.M. until 4:30 A.M. last night. She at first was very congested and then she started breathing with a groan every time she took a breath. We gave her some medicine for congestion and after about a half an hour, it started to work. We couldn't get a blood pressure off her right arm and we thought things were coming to an end. About 4:00 A.M., she started breathing more easier and we felt she was sleeping.

Today she has not hardly said a word. She does understand us, but her answer is more like a groan than a word.

I missed church today on Easter for the first time, I think, in my life. I was so tired; I was afraid I'd embarrass myself by falling a sleep in church.

The hospice nurse on call this weekend stopped by on the way to her church and dropped off some more medication. They are now just giving us a few days' supply at a time because it is so unusual for someone to hang on as long as Carol is doing. Forty-seven days without any nourishment is unbelievable.

Our kids, Robin and Bob, don't know what to do. Please pray for them.

God's will be done.

Bob

E-mails received Easter Sunday April 15:

Continuing to keep you in prayer, that you would find the strength to do the work that God has called you to do. We love you.

John & Sue

Thanks for keeping us aware of what is going on. You and Carol are in our prayers as you well know. I pray that you are taking care of yourself.

Hang in there and we will support you in any and all ways we can.

Dying with Carol

DeColores

Roger and Jeanette.

Robert,

I pray that God will give you wisdom. This must be incredibly difficult. May God bless your children with strength to get through this trial. In Christ's name AMEN.

Jesus is coming.

Brother Clayton
God's will be done

Monday April 16 e-mail from Bob:

We've been sitting at Carol's side all day waiting to see if she would take her last breath. This morning, our hospice nurse couldn't get a blood pressure and said her pulse was 160. There are also physical signs in her skin that the end is near. When the C.N.A. came to bath her she gave indication that she thought the end was near.

It's now 5:00 P.M. our time and Carol is still laboring with each breath. Her Good friend Jane is with her as I write this e-mail.

Keep praying that Carol finds her peace.

Today she said. "I want to die."

Bob

49 Days with Hospice

E-mails received April 16:

> We may not be there in person but we are there in spirit right beside you.
>
> God's peace to all of you.
>
> Mike and Ilona

> Dear Bob,
>
> All day today I felt that this could be the day she walks into Jesus' arms. What an emotional rest that would give you as I know you are concerned for her comfort and well being, but know you are exhausted (physically and emotionally). I leave for Florida Wed. and will not be back till the 29.
>
> Rog will give you a big hug from me when he sees you. God bless.
>
> Jeanette Kassing

Chapter 10

CAROL'S FUNERAL

Tuesday April 17 from Bob:

Carol went to be with our Lord at 2:00 P.M. today. She was surrounded by her brother, her sister-in law, and I.

Her are the particulars of her funeral:

Carol Lillie

Eureka, Ill. Carol Lillie of 205 Shady Lane died at her home on April 17, 2001 at 2:00 P.M.

Born August 20, 1935 to Frank and Margaret Blunier on a farm near Roanoke, Il.

She married Robert "Bob" Lillie on September 5, 1955. He survives. Also surviving are one son, Robert G. Lillie of Greenville, Indiana, and one daughter, Mrs. Robin

Dying with Carol

Crow of Phoenix, Arizona, and her brother, Cletus Blunier of Albuquerque, New Mexico.

She had two grandchildren. Her parents preceded her in death.

She graduated from Eureka High School and attended Illinois Central College and worked part time at local restaurants. She was locally known for her china painting talent.

She was a member of the Eureka United Methodist Church. She had served as a Stephen's minister for many years until her death. She was active in the Peoria Cursillo, The Walk to Emmaus where she was a lay director of Central Illinois Walk to Emmaus #99.

She was also active in Faith, Hope and Love's prison ministry and had served on teams at Dwight Correctional Center eleven times.

Visitation will be at the Argo, Rustman, Harris funeral Home in Eureka from 5 to 8 on Friday April 20.

The funeral service will be at the Eureka United Methodist Church at 11:00 A.M. on Saturday April 21. Rev. Scott Carlson will officiate.

Memorials can be made to her church, any Walk to Emmaus or Cursillo community.

Carol's Funeral

E-mails received after Carol's death:

Bob:

Obviously you have my condolences. I uttered a prayer of gratitude that Carol did not have to linger any longer, and then I asked God to comfort you.

I really want to help you out in any way I can. If we need to get together once in a while to just visit.

I don't think I have to tell you that you and Carol are dear to me. You have touched my life in more ways than you will ever know. You have both been Jesus with skin on to me many times over.

May God bless you and sustain you as you mourn the loss of a very special woman who was your best friend and lover.

Shalom,
Bruce

Bob and family,

I know that you will all miss Carol very much in the days-years ahead but for now I am praying that you will also rejoice in her victory over death.

If there is anything I can do for you, please let me know. You will remain in my prayers.

Pat Monroe

Dying with Carol

Dear Bob,

I am so sorry to hear about Carol's passing. As you have been saying, she is with the Lord. I hope that the few words from our liturgy can give you some small amount of consolation.

May the Angels take her into paradise
May The Martyrs come to Welcome her on her way
And lead her into the Holy City, Jerusalem.
May the choir of angels welcome her
And with Lazarus who once was poor
May she have everlasting rest.

Please know that you and your family have been and will always be in my prayers.

God loves you all, and so do I.

Bill Salz
Cursillo #606

Dear Ones;

Carol is now "perfection" with our Lord and Savior Jesus Christ! Hallelujah, Amen.

God Bless you and surround you in His perfect peace and mercy. Our hearts and prayers are as close as your breath.

With you in His love,
Lois

Carol's Funeral

Dear Robert,

God bless you and your family as He opens Heaven's Door for Carol.

You are in our thoughts and prayers, as always since Cursillo #606. Sorry we won't make it to her funeral.

Love,
Mark Seipel

Hi Bob;

Sorry to be writing at this time, but I just learned of Carol's illness yesterday, and her passing today from Bev Weber. You have been and will be in our prayers. If there is anything you need, please do not hesitate to call. We know that she is home with the Lord.

Sincerely,
David Lavallee
Music chair
Cursillo #606

Bob:

I cannot begin to tell you how sorry we are that Carol is gone. We will never understand why she spent the last 50 days unable to do anything. The joy in all this is that we all know she is now with our Heavenly Father. In that we must find the comfort we all need.

I am scheduled to bring you dinner on Friday. I want to do so as I know you will have a house full of people.

Dying with Carol

Larry will be home all day, so he can deliver it any time you want it. It will need to be warmed in the oven about 45 minutes. If you would like it early morning so you can eat whenever, just let us know. I want to help make Friday and Saturday as easy as possible for you and your family. I am so glad Cletus and Marty were there with you. I know how Bob and Robin must feel–but everyone knows the tough decisions one makes at a time like this. I was in the same situation and thanks to wonderful people like you and Carol, I was able to be with my Mother when she needed me.

I was called away suddenly just now–and told that another secretary had just passed away last night. No warning. We were planning lunch soon. How quickly our lives change. This has been a tough week.

My love to you and family. Let me know about Friday's meal.

In His love and mine,
Marsha

Bob,

Know that you continue to be in our prayers and thoughts. Sue will be here for the weekend so I am sure we will see you at that time. Know that you can call on us anytime and we will be there for you.

Blessings,
John and Sue

Carol's Funeral

Bob,

I just wanted you to know that I praise God for Carol and the wonderful witness that her life showed. I rejoice with you that she has gone on and is in God's loving arms. I also mourn with you and know that you will miss her. My prayers are with you and your family.

> God Bless,
> Pastor John M. Cross
> Sadorus/Parkville UMC

Bob, thank you for the beautiful photo of Carol. We pray that you are finding comfort in knowing that she is in a better place. I know that doesn't make missing her easier.

> Love,
> Virginia

Dear Bob & Family,

You have our deepest sympathy. I'm sure on one hand it is a blessing because you know Carol is at home finally, after all the suffering and yet we are sometimes selfish in letting loved ones go because we know they will be sadly missed.

We will be praying for comfort and peace for you and your family.

> Love,
> Kathern Mackay

Dying with Carol

Dear Bob,

Thank you for sharing the picture of Carol–it was beautiful! She was beautiful!

Thank you, also, for sharing your e-mails the past several months. They were personal witnesses to your love for Carol and faith in Jesus. We have been blessed to know you both, and to share this part of your faith journey together.

Carol reached home before us. I wonder if she's planting a garden in heaven?! We'll see.

Love,
Huck, Dalene
and Family

Amen. We don't know you folks well–just Emmaus friends–but have followed your trials all along. What an inspiration you are to all! I know you will miss Carol but your faith has certainly carried you through this so beautifully. I know you will face some difficult times but God has been with you all this time and will continue to be with you until you are reunited with Carol in His home! God bless you!

Dear Bob;

I expected to be able to attend either the visitation or funeral but am assigned as hospital chaplain in Rushville this week until Sunday morning. Just know that Carolyn and I will continue to keep you and the family in prayer during this difficult time.

Carol's Funeral

We love you Bob and know that we will all see Carol again because of the reality of the resurrection.

Peace to you my dear friend.

Carl Wiggins

Bob, I want you to know that I am very proud to have been a part of your love story with Carol over the past several months. The love that you showed and that you relayed through your daily sharing has touched me very much. I always looked forward to your updates so I could witness this great gift that you shared in those final days. I'm sure you miss Carol very much but I know that you let her go to God because that is what we all are striving for. You have been in my thoughts and prayers these past months and I thank you for making me a part of it. The strength that you displayed in your faith and in your love of God truly is a gift from God. I always remember that God doesn't give us more than we can handle and I just witnessed that these past several weeks. I'm sure you may have questioned your strength a time or two but from this view it was always strong and you accepted that God was in charge.

I'm sorry for your loss and I will say a special prayer that Carol is at peace with our Lord and that you are at peace knowing that is true.

God Bless,
Tim Conklin

Dying with Carol

Just a note to let you know that my Group Reunion said a prayer for you last Monday as we closed. We lauded your commitment to the Lord and to Carol.

I went to Mass this morning at Sacred Heart in Peoria and again my thoughts were of you. May He continue to bless you and hold you in the palm of His hand.

Jim Behme

Excerpts from Scott Carson's funeral service for Carol:

This morning we welcome you to this special service in celebration of this Christian life of Carol Lillie.

Friends, we have gathered here to praise God, to witness to our faith as we celebrate the life of Carol Lillie. Carol was born on August the 20, 1935 the daughter of Frank and Margaret Blunier on a farm near Roanoke. She died this Tuesday, April 17 at her home in Eureka. Carol and Bob were married on September 4, 1955, here in the church sanctuary.

Carol was known for her beautiful work with china painting porcelain, many of these pieces are in their living room at home, and many of you as family and friends were given a piece of her work over the last years.

She was a homemaker, a wife, a mother, a Christian woman. She was active and a dedicated part of this church.

Carol's Funeral

Carol passed from this life to her place our Heavenly father prepared for her in one of her favorite times of the year, spring. She loved flowers, daffodils, and narcissi, tulips, and the hyacinth that were coming up in the yard and around the driveway.

She loved the birds and she would often sit in the kitchen and watch them to make sure Bob kept the bird feeder full. Before long the hummingbirds would be coming back which she really liked, and her rose bushes would be budding and blooming for their most beautiful blooms.

There is so much to lift up about Carol in this short time, we cannot adequately mention all the ways that God blessed her, or the ways that she blessed other people.

One of the very special things about Carol and Bob for that matter was their love for other people. We know from scripture that the greatest of all Christian things is love.

Carol deeply loved people; she loved to have others as her friend and she loved being a friend. Friendship was one of her special gifts.

Someone has said when we are young in years, that is when we are young people, we have all of the time and few memories, and when we are older, we have all of the memories, but little time.

Carol thoroughly enjoyed the passage of time. She especially enjoyed the gift of Christian friendship.

Dying with Carol

Some of you even in your deep, deep loss today know that you have been uniquely blessed to have had Carol Lillie as your friend and you will never be the same because of her friendship. Your life from this point on will always be different and better and enriched because she was your friend.

I think you know how grateful Carol was for those of you who were her friends, and those of you who cared for her these last many months in the hospital and in the home. People from hospice also cared for her in special and wonderful ways.

Carol also lived an exemplary and spiritual life. Carol was not haughty, nor did she ever seek credit, that I was aware of. She lived the humble values of the new kingdom, not the earthly kingdom, but the kingdom of God.

Just before we came in here, the immediate family and I had a prayer in the prayer chapel here where Carol so deeply loved praying with her Emmaus group every Sunday. She loved Sunday school and worship, and prayer, and receiving Holy Communion.

You can tell a lot about a person from their Bible. To say that it is a well worn and used book is an understatement. It is filled with all kinds of special things Carol has collected over a lifetime of faith.

There's a beautiful inscription, really two beautiful inscriptions, from Bob, who gave the Bible to Carol.

Carol loved and enjoyed fellowship with Jesus Christ, her living Lord and Savior.

Carol's Funeral

Carol and Bob have also been a spiritual example in terms of marriage and the family.

Prior to this past Christmas, Carol was thoroughly enjoying the preparation she was doing for the arrival for her children and her grandchildren.

Then when Christmas time came when all those children and grandchildren were here, she was totally in her glory. Some of those of us around her just sensed the glory and when they all came to church that Sunday we celebrated with her.

Carol and Bob were an example of Christian marriage. They had forty-five tears of marriage and in September it would have been forty-six.

They often spoke words of love and appreciation to each other. They treated each other kindly. They were spiritual friends. We are so grateful for their example.
And lastly, Carol extended the Kingdom of God to other people. Carol extended the Kingdom of God through Stephen's Ministry. Her Care-receiver so wanted to be here this morning, but was unable to.

Through Emmaus, she directed Walk number 99.

Some of Carol's close special friends, are not here as they are preparing for another Emmaus event. They are holding a memorial service today for Carol at the retreat center.

Dying with Carol

She was active with Faith, Hope, and Love, prison ministries based in Peoria and she made at least eleven trips to Dwight Correctional Center.

Carol had a tremendous heart for women prisoners, and they deeply loved her. One of the stories that I heard that I thought was precious, about Carol and her work at Dwight Correctional Center. Something that sometimes she did repeatedly, she wasn't supposed to do, but she did it anyway. You can't take any photographs into the prison at all. Carol routinely smuggled photographs into prison and it amazing what she took into prison for the women, who would sit around those tables with her. She would show them picture of (do you know what it is?) her flowers. And they would hover around her and they would look at those pictures and they would oo and ah, because they knew that was one of the things most beautiful and she was sharing something so deeply personal of herself. They were also thinking about someday in the future when they might be able to go home and have flowers. She touched the women deeply at Dwight.

Carol also extended the Kingdom of God every Sunday morning in the church foyer. Pastors know you can never replace people. We hope that some of you take up her ministry of welcoming people in the foyer whether you were a new member or just a visitor, or an old friend.

You know what I'm speaking about. She went from person to person and just greeted and welcomed, and encouraged people in their faith and she extended the Kingdom of God in that wonderful practical way. She truly enjoyed Christian fellowship.

Today we celebrate this special Christian life. Each of you can take something in your heart to remind in ways she has so deeply enriched you in Christian faith and fellowship.

We are grateful to God, amen.

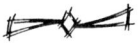

At this point, I think, I had better sum up why I compiled this narrative.

Throughout this time of Carol's dying, I shared what I was going through with the Body of Christ, that make up my Christian friends. Without their prayers and support, I don't think I would have been able to come through these times.

Carol did die, I think as you read the series of daily e-mails, you could sense the change that came on me from praying for a complete recovery to praying for more time with her, to the final stage where I prayed that God would take her home.

These are stages of dying that I went through during the months from September 2000 until April 17, 2001.
I can't say that I experienced the stage of anger that some people go through in the process of accepting the death of a loved one. I may have been unhappy with one of

the nurses during the hospital stay, but that was only a very temporary thing.

What I did really experience is the love of hundreds of fellow Christians who were praying for us and loving us during this time.

This is the reason for writing this narrative. To let others know that the Body of Christ is alive and well, especially in the Cursillo, Walk to Emmaus, and my local United Methodist church.

As Carol said early in this dying experience, "I don't know how anyone could face this without a strong belief in a Loving God."

Amen to that.

Chapter 11

BOB'S THANK YOU SERMON

On Sunday, July 15 2001, I was asked to fill the pulpit for Scott Carlson. My talk was, "The Body Of Christ."

The Body of Christ

As many of you know, the last eight months have been very trying in my life. One thing that has become very clear to me over this time was that my family was far more than just the people who were related to me by blood or marriage.

From the time of the early Christian church, the followers of Jesus were first called the church and then the Body of Christ as you heard in today's scripture, (1 Corinthians 12:27).

Today when we say the word "church" most people thing about a building such as our United Methodist Church, here in Eureka to the huge Basilica of St. Peter's in Rome. But in the first century of Christianity, the term church was used for the people of Jesus. For the most part, they met in private homes because they were not permitted to meet in the synagogues.

After Pentecost, when the Holy Spirit descended on the disciples and others followers of Jesus, they knew that the Spirit of God actually inhabited the bodies of the people and the term Body of Christ became synonymous for the people of God.

During these last months when we found out that Carol first had the beginning stages of breast cancer and then advanced indications of ovarian cancer, The Body of Christ (the people of God) became far more important to me.

God's grace comes in many forms. Most of the time, we find it in our belief that we are saved or justified because of Jesus' death on the cross which paid the price for our sins.

God, however, uses the people of God to act as his hands in this world.

We are and can be God's instruments in this world.

In his book, *That man is you*, Louis Evely puts it this way.

> Lay people, by and large, underestimate their vocation. They don't understand their vocation. They don't understand that God needs them right where they are to carry on His work among men, that He is counting on them to perfect and sanctify the world; they don't realize that he's committed this task, this business, these children, this man and this woman to them, and that we're all like the wise and prudent manager who's been put in charge of some of his Master's goods and servants in order to give each one what he needs when he needs it.

Bob's Thank You Sermon

Let's look at it this way: God needed someone, where we are now, to guide this child, to comfort this man or woman, to perform this job, to prove His love.

Couldn't he have done that all himself, without relying on us? Yes, God could've done everything, all by Himself, but he so made the world that things wouldn't be as good that way.

He chose to need men; He's willed that we be necessary to him, for the fulfillment of his design.

"You'll do greater deeds than I."

He's permanently set up the universe is such a way, that God with man can accomplish more than God alone . . ."

(*That man is you*, Louis Evely; translated by Edmond Bonin, © 1964, Paulist Press, New York, Ramsey, Toronto, pages 206–208.)

This is where I was the beneficiary of God's grace through the Body of Christ that makes up this church and other Christian friends.

On October 3, when Carol had her first of two surgeries for breast cancer and ovarian cancer, besides Scott, the waiting room was filled with our son and his wife, our daughter, my niece Tammy, Elton and Joyce Lanier, Rog and Jane Griffith from this church, several of Robin's friends, one drove all the way from Dekalb, Robin's in-laws from Delavan, and several other friends that we have made through the Walk to Emmaus.

I was surrounded by the Body of Christ during Carol's surgery.

Dying with Carol

I also did something I had never done before and that was ask for prayers for ourselves.

I don't know what it is about we Christians, but we have no qualms about praying for someone else, but we are reluctant to ask for prayers for ourselves.

Many of us are good givers, but we are reluctant receivers.

Maybe that is why we find it hard to understand that God's grace is an undeserved gift, and that we are saved because of what Jesus did for us, not because of what we may have done. We seem reluctant to except the free gift from God.

I don't know if it's pride (which is a sin) or the feeling of unworthiness (which is one of the devil's tools), but something in us seems to make us reluctant to ask God for things for ourselves.

I just finished a small book by Bruce Wilkinson called, *The Prayer of Jabez*. It's about a short prayer you can find in the Old Testament in 1 Chronicles 4:10.

It is noteworthy, because in this short prayer Jabez asks God for things for himself.

"Oh, that You would bless me indeed and enlarge my territory, that Your hand would be with me and that You would keep me from evil, that I may not cause pain!"

The verse goes on, "So God granted him what he had requested."

We should pray for ourselves. Not just when your back is against the wall and the lady who you spent 45 years with is in the hands of doctors, and there is nothing you can personally do, and you are forced to drop your armor and ask for prayers.

Bob's Thank You Sermon

I started during this time and until Carol died on April 17, to send out e-mail requests for prayers. Many of you in this church whose e-mail address I had, received them, and many of the people I knew through Cursillo and the Walk to Emmaus received them also.

Originally, I was sending out about sixty e-mails a day, but another wonderful thing happened. Many of the people who received these e-mails passed them on to their friends, most of whom we didn't know.

Those who sent prayers back to me, I added to my list which eventually grew to 96 e-mails a day, I was sending out.

God was expanding my territory.

As I said many people responded back to me with prayers and encouragement. By the time Carol died, we had over 700 replies and prayers from all over the country.

An example of this is:

Dear Mr. Lillie,

I just wanted to assure you and your wife of my prayers as she undergoes surgery tomorrow. May the God of Grace, the colors of which have shown so brightly, through her involvement in Cursillo and Emmaus, shine brighter in the recovery and healing God brings.

Please know of my concern and desire for an update as you have the opportunity.

In Christ,
Ron Colwell, Director
The Upper Room Emmaus

Dying with Carol

Our prayers were answered during the surgery and Carol did come through it all right. We were told that surgery could not remove all of her ovarian cancer, but we were given a hope that chemotherapy might possibly bring a cure or at least a remission.

Carol was able to come home from the hospital and spend some quality time at home.

She even had a mother's dream, where both of our children and all of our grandchildren were at our house for Christmas.

After the first of the year, we resumed the chemotherapy and Carol began to have some ill effects from the treatment. By the end of January she had stopped eating and about the first of February, she again entered the hospital and on Sunday February 3, she had emergency surgery for a bowel blockage.

She came through that surgery all right, but the next day she had what we now think was a mild stroke. This made it impossible for her to swallow or eat.

Throughout this time, we kept receiving e-mails.

On February 8, I received this one:

> Carol has really been through it all this past year and still, I will be praying for her. Bob, we all know God does answer prayer, and how are you holding up thru all of this? You too are in my prayers, so that God will touch you both, comfort you and give you peace.
>
> Love,
> Kathern

Bob's Thank You Sermon

And on February 9 we received another note:

Dear Bob,

Just wanted you to know that you and Carol were lifted up in prayer at 1st United Methodist Church choir in Peoria tonight. You must be exhausted beyond belief,

With love,
Jannette and Roger Kassing

I won't try to read them all as I told you we have received over 700 e-mails, but you get the idea of how the Body of Christ supported us throughout this period.

Carol came home with hospice on February 28. It was determined that because of her inability to swallow that prolonging her life by artificial means was not the way she wanted to live.

When we brought her home both the doctor and hospice told us they didn't believe that Carol would last over three or four days.

It was during this time that my e-mails changed. I was no longer asking for Carol's healing from cancer. I was now asking that God's will be done and that she not experience any pain.

When we say the Lord's Prayer, we say, "Thy kingdom come, Thy will be done." How many times have I prayed that, but was really asking for my will to be done.

During the next 49 days that Carol held on without any nourishment, I truly, in my heart, was asking for God's will to be done. My prayers were answered. Carol, throughout these days, did not experience pain from the cancer, although there were signs that it was growing again.

E-mail after e-mail came in from all across the country from many from you. I truly felt the prayers and support of what we call the Body of Christ.

Toward the end Carol had lost so much weight that she began to remind of the young bride I had married 45 years ago.

Scott was almost a daily visitor during these days as well as her many friends in this church. Carolyn came and sang for her. Krista Brockman came and talked to her about heaven.

Sue Ewan drove all the way from Missouri while Carol was still in the hospital to help prepare her and to tell Carol it was all right to go.

Never in my life have I felt the power of God's grace so alive in the people who make up our portion of the Body of Christ.

Do I miss her?

You bet I do!

But I know that I am not alone.

I'm surrounded by a loving church, the Body of Christ here in Eureka, and a loving Christian community around the State of Illinois and the world known **as the** Cursillo and Walk to Emmaus.

Would you join me in prayer.

To order additional copies of

DYING WITH CAROL

Have your credit card ready and call:

1-877-421-READ (7323)

or please visit our web site at
www.pleasantword.com

Also available at: www.amazon.com

NOTE FROM THE AUTHOR

About a year and a half after Carol died my daughter, who lives in Phoenix, AZ. convinced me that it would be easier on her if I finished out what years I might have left closer to her than the 1700 miles which separated us during her mother's illness.

In the course of moving, I lost the e-mail addresses that I communicated with during the time frame of this book.

Would anyone who reads this book who was receiving the e-mail letters please contact me. Also, anyone who reads this book who would like to respond to me please feel free to do so. My e-mail address is: rclillie@cox.net

Printed in the United States
1448100002B/1-66